W9-BIB-606

"The US health care system is broken," Joshua Freemen tells us in the opening line of his powerful critique, *Health, Medicine and Justice: Designing a Fair and Equitable Healthcare System.* He spends the next 300 pages masterfully and persuasively documenting this charge. His voice is disappointed more than it is angry or shrill. Freeman is a practicing family physician and the chairman of the Department of Family Medicine at the University of Kansas School of Medicine. It is his system and he wants to see it perform as it should, to work in a more equitable fashion, and to produce results that the country is paying for but not getting. His command of fact is impressive and his tone caring and therapeutic. He tells us about everything from comparative health systems in Europe to profit motives in the Board Room. Dr. Freeman concludes that a single payer health system is the solution to better and more equitable healthcare in America. It is "political will," he tells us, "that will fix the broken system."

—Fitzhugh Mullan, M.D.
Murdock Head Professor of Medicine and Health Policy,
Professor of Pediatrics The George Washington University

"In his book, *Health, Medicine and Justice*, Joshua Freeman not only explains the unique features of the U.S. health care system that result in significantly higher costs but only mediocrity in performance, he also discusses the issues against a background of health care justice. This leads to the compelling conclusion that, being all in this together, we can apply principles of health care justice to ensure higher quality health care for everyone, at a level of spending that the nation can afford."

—Don McCanne, M.D., Senior Health Policy Fellow,
Physicians For a National Health Program (PNHP)

"This is an informative and entertaining overview of the current status and deficiencies of the US healthcare system. It will serve as a useful text for anyone just beginning their inquiry into how the system works, or for someone wanting a refresher course on the influences of social policy and values on the outcomes of the unique approaches to providing healthcare prevalent in the US."

—Robert Graham, M.D., former CEO,
American Academy of Family Physicians

"Whether simplifying the arcane methods of financing graduate medical education, or clarifying the inaccuracies and conflicts of interest in the way that medical schools report their production of primary care doctors, Dr Freeman provides insight into the bases for our out-of-balance health care workforce. In an engaging and understandable style, he not only identifies the underlying issues but also points to some opportunities for righting the health care system's deficiencies; and makes a strong argument for why we should do so. If you don't care about social justice and don't want to risk caring more, don't read this book."

—Christine C. Matson M.D., Glenn Mitchell Chair
in Generalist Medicine; Chair, Department of Family and
Community Medicine, Eastern Virginia Medical School

"Dr. Freeman covers a wide landscape related to the key issues of health care delivery and quality. Underlying his progressive analysis and solutions is a humane family medicine perspective. He puts it together in a way that draws lasting lessons—re-educate trainees to think and practice differently, change the system to make appropriate care the norm, and reorganize health care financing to move toward a true universal health care system."

—Mardge Cohen, M.D., WE-ACTx, Rwanda,
and Boston Health Care for the Homeless

HEALTH, MEDICINE AND JUSTICE

*Designing a Fair and Equitable
Healthcare System*

Joshua Freeman, M.D.

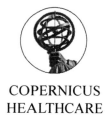

COPERNICUS
HEALTHCARE

Health, Medicine and Justice
Designing a Fair and Equitable Healthcare System

Joshua Freeman, M.D.

Copernicus Healthcare
Friday Harbor, WA

First Edition
Copyright ©2015 by Joshua Freeman, M.D. All rights reserved

Book design, cover and illustrations by W. Bruce Conway

No portion of this work may be reproduced or transmitted in any form or by any means, electronic or mechanical, including photocopying and recording, or by an information storage or retrieval system, without written permission from the publisher.

softcover: ISBN 978-0-9887996-8-4

Library of Congress Control Number: 2014957664

Copernicus Healthcare
34 Oak Hill Drive
Friday Harbor, WA 98250

www.copernicus-healthcare.org

Contents

Tables and Figures

Acknowledgements

I first must thank two incredibly important people to me, who ensure that discussion of ideas is valued and application is possible; that practice (experience) and theory are combined into meaningful praxis:

Patricia Kelly for her wisdom, guidance, feedback and support through this entire process.

Adam Freeman for his ideas, insight, and feedback, and being a great mind to discuss health policy (and virtually anything else!)

I thank Esther Fernandez for her tireless work in putting together materials and making this possible.

Finally, I thank the University of Kansas School of Medicine, which provided me with the sabbatical in which the bulk of this book was written. The facts are the facts, but the opinions expressed are mine alone, and do not reflect those of the University of Kansas, the University of Kansas Medical Center, or the School of Medicine.

Preface

While out of town over Thanksgiving in 2008, shortly after the election of President Obama, I decided to create a blog. I am not sure why; maybe I had been reading about blogs, and wondered if it was really as easy as it seemed to just create a site on the Internet to share ones thoughts. It turned out to be quite easy, and I soon had created a blog, *Medicine and Social Justice*. The title simply combined two areas that I knew something about and thought I had something to offer anyone who might find their way to it. My first post, on November 28, 2008, reflected on an article in *The Nation* by Alexander Cockburn, and on the creation of the Kansas Health Policy Authority by Governor Sebelius—now defunct, by decision of Governor Brownback. But mostly it talked about the need for a universal health coverage plan; near the end I put *Cover Everybody!* in bold italics, and ended with an idea for a bumper sticker: *If you don't think we need a program to provide health coverage to everyone, it's ok. We can leave you out!*

In some ways, that first blog was a "gimme", calling for a universal, single-payer health system as I had for many years, along with many others in this country, in particular Physicians for a National Health Program (PNHP). The next day I took a completely different tack with "Mumbai, Valley Stream, and the Economic Meltdown", counterposing the terrorist attack in India's largest city with the financial crisis we had recently begun and a much less-well-remembered event, the trampling to

1

death of a young Wal-Mart worker named Jdimytai Damour as "Black Friday" crowds stormed into the store looking for things that they could still afford. Nothing about health care; this early on I had not decided necessarily to write about *both* medicine *and* social justice in each blog post. Indeed, my third post (on the third day—I was doing them daily!) was about both in a very sad way, acknowledging the death of Steven Tamarin, M.D., a family physician from New York City who was deeply committed to both issues, and who I knew from our joint service on the board of directors of Physicians for Reproductive Choice and Health (PRCH), now Physicians for Reproductive Health (PRH).

I continued regular posting for the rest of that month, undoubtedly facilitated by the holidays, with 16 posts by the end of the year. As I got more practiced, I began to develop a style. I also began to post a little less often, 2-3 times a week instead of daily. I focused on issues that were important to me, many of them things I had thought about for a long time and now took advantage of a place to say them. I also decided to base the posts on one or more articles that had appeared in the medical literature (frequently *JAMA,* the *New England Journal of Medicine,* and *Health Affairs*) or in coverage by major news outlets, most often the *New York Times.* This has continued as I have continued the blog, generally once a week. I look for articles in the medical literature that are important but do not seem to be getting adequate coverage or for which the coverage is confusing and sometimes simplistic. I try to address my writing to what I think of as "educated laypersons." I assume significant general literacy, but do not assume *medical* literacy, as my experience has been that very smart and well-educated people expert in their own fields often do not understand what I take to be basic concepts of medicine and health care (just as I understand almost nothing about engineering).

I have thought for some time about writing a book that addresses many of these themes in a single volume. The University of Kansas School of Medicine, my employer, approved a sabbatical for me, with this book as a primary project. This book is not a compendium of blogs, although it draws heavily from them, and often reproduces parts of them verbatim. Clearly, over the years, many of the things I have written about are dated, so it does not attempt to address all of them. Also, there are excellent books that address many of these themes, some of which I have included as references in the chapters and the final bibliography [e.g., Donohoe's *Public Health and Social Justice,* Farmer works, several Geyman books, Richard Young's *American Health Scare* and the 2002 book of essays on *Medicine and Social Justice]*. I hope that this book complements the others, offering a perspective that combines a physician's knowledge of medical care and how it is delivered, a scholar's understanding of the organization of the health system, social determinants of health and health disparities, a caring person's commitment to justice and equity, and an activist's desire to change the world. I hope it is of some value.

CHAPTER 1

Why Do We Have
A Healthcare System?

"Every system is perfectly designed to get the results that it gets."

—Paul Batalden, MD[1]

The U.S. health care system is broken. People are dying prematurely, they are suffering with ill health before they die, they are unable to access care when they need it. We are inundated with expensive, high-technology, specialist-driven care, much of it occurring at the end of life, but we do not have nearly enough primary care to help prevent illness, or diagnose and treat it early in its course. We do very little to address the social conditions in which people live that are largely responsible for poor health. We educate our future physicians in the rarefied atmosphere of academic medical centers, where uncommon conditions are the norm and common conditions, when they are seen, are in their end stages. Our health outcomes are abysmal when compared to other industrialized countries. Our media hype every new scientific breakthrough, and we spend a great deal on medical research, but we don't do well applying it. In fact, we do a very poor job of providing the care that we already know how to do in order to improve people's health.

It's not for lack of money. The U.S. spends far more, overall and *per capita* on "health care," than any other country in the world, including all those whose health status is far better than ours. The amount of money spent *per capita* should be buying us superb health, but it isn't. The 2013 report from the distinguished Institute of Medicine (IOM) of the National Academy of Sciences, aptly titled "Shorter Lives, Poorer Health"[2] provides extensive documentation of the U.S. health disadvantage compared to our peers. Of the 17 richest countries,* the U.S. is 14 is mortality from communicable disease, 16 in mortality from non-communicable disease, and 16 in mortality from injuries—and no country is below us in more than one category. Our mortality rates from major causes of death are above the 17-nation average for 15 conditions and at or below the average for only 6.

Our life expectancy at birth is last for males and next-to-last for females. We have the lowest probability of survival to age 50, and at no age until 75 is our life expectancy higher than #15. While our infant mortality rates have continued to drop, we have not kept pace with these other countries; not only are our rates 17th in this group but are 31st among all members of the Organization for Economic Cooperation and Development (OECD). There are certain areas where we are outstandingly bad: obesity, motor vehicle fatalities, and of course gun violence. In 2007, 69% of U.S. homicides (73% of homicides before age 50) involved firearms, compared with 26% in peer countries; a 2003 study found that the U.S. homicide rate was 7 times higher (the rate of firearm homicides was 20 times higher) than in 22 OECD countries, and

---

* Australia, Austria, Canada, Denmark, Finland, France, Germany, Italy, Japan, Norway, Portugal, Spain, Sweden, Switzerland, The Netherlands, United Kingdom, United States

although U.S. suicide rates were lower than in those countries, firearm suicide rates were 6 times higher.

Some have suggested this reflects the diversity of U.S. society, in particular that we have a large number of minority groups. While I cannot imagine how this would be in any way a justification, the fact remains that if we consider only non-Hispanic whites, our mortality rates below the age of 55 are never better than 16th, for either sex. Our infant mortality rates for both non-Hispanic whites and mothers with over 16 years of education are also higher than other countries.[3]

Our only real lead, as noted above, is in cost. U.S. healthcare spending is about $8,000 per capita per year, while the other 16 countries spend between $2,500 and $5,000. Mapping life expectancy against spending, as in Figure 1.1, should embarrass us all. Despite all the money we spend, our life expectancy is not only below that of the other 16 countries, it exceeds that of only a few OECD countries, all spending less than $2,000 per capita per year.

Given the data, it is hard to argue that the system is not broken, and this has led to many efforts to "fix" it. The most prominent recent example, of course, is the Affordable Care Act (popularly known as Obamacare), passed in 2010 and implemented in 2013 and 2014. Like Medicare and Medicaid nearly 50 years earlier, the ACA has had a major impact, allowing many who were previously uninsured, or uninsurable because of pre-existing conditions, to gain coverage. But it still does not ensure coverage for everyone, and by using the private insurance system (unlike Medicare) it does ensure continued high cost. Nor have we yet seen a significant effort to increase the number of primary care physicians (or other providers), and worse, rather than addressing the social determinants of health, we have continued to decimate

Figure 1.1

Large Differences in Life Expectancy and Health Care Spending Across OECD Countries

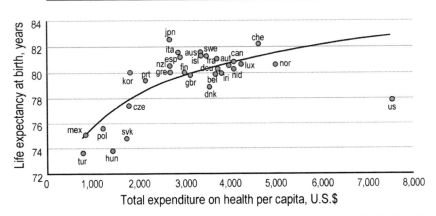

Source: OECD Health Data 2010. Available at: http://www.oecd.org/eco/growth/46508904.pdf

the social support systems that are necessary for health and continued to move almost all "health care" funding into medical care.

The real issue is "what are we trying to achieve?" What is the goal of our healthcare system? Batalden's Law, cited earlier, that every system is perfectly designed to get the results that it gets, is obviously true. This means that the problem isn't that our system is not working, but that it is working just fine to achieve the wrong goals. We are getting what our system is it is designed to get—profit and wealth for those who control it, rather than health for the people of the nation.

Starting with the principles that guide us, health, health care, medical care, and the organization of our health system are integrally tied to issues of justice and equity. A big part of having a system that is focused on making money rather than on health is that it is unjust and inequitable, both by not providing necessary health care to those who need it and by providing unnecessary care to those who do not. We must create a just and equitable system that reverses this. It should provide everyone with the health care they need while removing wasteful care. It must eliminate incentives for delivering unneeded care and be organized in favor of providing what people do need to everyone who needs it. Its actions must grow from a scope that encompasses the core social determinants of health, and it must increase the focus on prevention.

The results that we get are designed into the system. These include: wasteful spending (more than any other country) that provides worse care; a focus on delivering profits over health care that matters; a focus on training too many subspecialists and then rewarding them in ways that devalues and limits the delivery of primary care; a research infrastructure focused on profit over public health; and a delivery system geared to treating people based on their wealth, not their health.

Batalden's Law is obvious if you think about it, but we often do not think about it. When we have results that are so unjust, where so many people are unnecessarily suffering and some are dying, where there is not justice, where there is not equity, we might wonder how we could have designed a system so poorly. Part of the answer, of course, is that it was not explicitly designed; it grew, and it grew in response to forces that are not about justice, not about equity, and not always or even mostly about health for our entire population. It should be.

There is a story widely recounted, much more often in schools of public health than in medical schools.

Once upon a time a man fishing in a river saw a body floating by. He pulled it out, but then saw another coming down-

stream. As he pulled that one out, he saw two more coming, then more after that. He called for help. People came to help. But the bodies kept coming faster and faster. People organized brigades, and used all available technology, building a conveyer belt to bring the bodies to a safe spot and digging mass graves. It was very efficient, but the bodies kept coming. Finally, someone said, "You know, maybe we should go upstream and find out what's killing these people...."

The story is a good illustration of our health system. We are willing to spend enormous sums of money to pull the bodies out of the river, but very little on preventing them from falling in. We need to not only identify *why* people are dying, but intervene to prevent them from dying by keeping them healthy in the first place. Inverting Batalden's Law, we need to be clear about the results that we want to have and build a system designed to achieve them, rather than tinkering with a deeply flawed system that was designed to achieve the wrong ends, and hoping for the best.

This is a theme I will come back to in several chapters, on issues including characteristics of the health workforce and the medical education experience: *first* it is necessary to decide what our outcomes should be (What should be people's health status? Just how many bodies floating down the river, "stupid deaths," as Paul Farmer calls them, should we tolerate?)[4] *Then*, with those outcomes in mind, we should design the best system that we can to achieve them.

I believe we can have a healthier society. We can have a health system based upon health for all people, not a few or some, and not about the profit that can be made from it. We can have a society and a healthcare system that is more just, that significantly decreases or eliminates inequities in health. We can have a health workforce that is made up of people with the right skill set needed to meet our healthcare needs. We can have a medical education system that is designed with that same outcome as its goal. We can have scientific and technological advances that create the opportunity for longer productive lives without sacrificing our ability to care about people as individuals and as a group. We can have a healthcare system that creates *value*, that doesn't spend so much money for second-class outcomes, and we can do it if we base it in *values*, values of health, and justice, and equity, while eschewing venality, narrowness and selfishness.

We can have all of this, but getting there will not be easy. It will mean changing a system that is entrenched, and often based on assumptions that are widely accepted, even when they are wrong. It will mean threatening, to a degree at least, the wealth and power and privilege of a small group in the interests of all of us. The recent passage and implementation of the Affordable Care Act provides an excellent object lesson. Despite being based on a model created by a conservative think tank (the Heritage Foundation) and despite being modeled on a state-wide program put in place in Massachusetts by Republican Governor (and 2012 presidential candidate) Mitt Romney, and despite providing enormous amounts of money to private insurance companies, it has been subject to constant attack, dozens of votes in the House to repeal it, and an inaccurate and irrational perception of it among much of the public.

The ACA, however, is in place. Millions of Americans who were previously uninsured now have health coverage. In this sense, it is the greatest victory since the passage of Medicare and Medicaid under President Johnson in the 1960s. It will no longer be possible to deny people insurance coverage because they are sick, and although those who do not have employer-based coverage will be required to buy individual policies, there will be federal subsidies for many who cannot afford it. Young people, who are finding it increasingly hard to get into the workforce, will be able to stay on their parents' insurance.

But even with these real successes, and despite the chorus of attacks from those who think it has done too much, the ACA will not solve our healthcare problems or lead us to a just and equitable society. Millions of people that the law intended to be covered by an expansion of the Medicaid program will not be, because the Supreme Court decision allowed states to opt out, and about half of the states have. This means many of the poorest and most needy will remain without health insurance, an outcome far removed from the principle of justice. The law does not cover those who are in this country without legal documentation, a politically popular decision, perhaps, but one that leaves many millions of people who are here, who are working and contributing, and who do get sick, without coverage. The enormous amounts of federal money being poured into the coffers of private insurance companies in order for them to support the ACA ensure that we will continue to be the nation that spends the most per capita on health care, even while excluding those millions of people. This continued waste means that the basic social needs of people, needs that have a profound impact on our health as a nation, including housing, food, and education, will continue to go unaddressed for lack of money.

The topics covered in this book all are related to justice, and to health, and to how health is a measure of how just our society is, and how a well-thought-out and designed health system can contribute to improving that. How, then, do justice and health interact?

Justice, Equity and Health

We most often think of "justice" in terms of the legal system, epitomized by a blind goddess holding a scale—and often a sword. In this sense, justice is seen by many as punishment for crimes or transgressions Justice, however, is a core measure of all aspects of a society; in health and in all social goods it is a question of access, fairness and the type of society we want to live in. It is about identifying how we can best meet the health needs of most people.

Justice in health care refers to the concept that people with the same conditions should have the same treatments available. It is intrinsic to medicine, and indeed is one of the four foundational principles of medical ethics, along with beneficence (and its partner, non-maleficence), and autonomy.[5] In my experience, however, and reflected by Darrell Kirch and David Vernon writing in *JAMA* in 2009, justice is one of principles least discussed in medical education or, indeed, in decisions being made in patient care settings, even when they involve ethics consultants. Teachers who lead ethics discussion groups of medical students often hear them discuss the relative importance, and the potentially conflicting implications, of "non-maleficence" (do no wrong) and "autonomy", as, for instance, when a person wishes a costly intervention that physicians believe will not help and may hurt. Justice does not mean that everyone, or even those with the same condition, should have the same treatment, because there are other factors (including individual preference) that impact the choice of treatment. It does mean that the options for those treatments should be available to all. In this sense, the "justice" of medical ethics is a subset of social justice, or distributive justice. Kirch and Vernon conclude that:

> *Physicians have a responsibility to ask and answer these difficult questions that are properly viewed as not simply involving politics, but rather as speaking to fundamental medical ethics. The answers in turn may well require personal sacrifices (eg, accepting a lower level of income), professional group action (eg, advocating as much for health care system improvements as current advocacy for the preservation of specialty reimbursement levels), and a commitment to work within the political process (that goes beyond lobbying for maintenance of the status quo). These efforts and corresponding sacrifices are necessary first steps toward creating a society in which everyone has access to appropriate health care.*[6]

The term "social justice", now widely used, particularly by many religious groups, was popularized by the philosopher John Rawls in the 1970s, although obviously the concept has been in existence, in one form or another, for centuries. In *A Theory of Justice*, Rawls writes:

> *All social primary goods—liberty and opportunity, income and wealth, and the bases of self-respect—are to be distributed equally unless an unequal distribution of any or all of these goods is to the advantage of the least favored.*[7]

"Distributed equally" is expansive, but the inclusion of the phrase "to the advantage of the least favored" suggests that things are not completely equal because there *are* least favored. For example, even in a much more equal society than we have, some people will suffer from physical or mental challenges that require them to utilize more resources.

A few decades before Rawls, Franklin Roosevelt said that "The test of our progress is not whether we add more to the abundance of those who have much; it is whether we provide enough to those who have too little." [8] This does not suggest that everything be divided equally, but makes a different moral claim: that what we as a society (and here we can read "government") should do is to help those who need the help most rather than those who need it the least. Throughout history, including today, that concept has been rejected by many. In any case it is clear that, today in the U.S., we do not have a system of social justice such as that described by either Rawls or Roosevelt; rather we have a system in which the most privileged exert great influence, and consistently use it to increase their privilege.

A concept closely related to social justice is that of human rights. The most authoritative modern definition is that of the *UN Universal Declaration of Human Rights*, passed in 1948. Article 25 states that:

Everyone has the right to a standard of living adequate for the health and well-being of himself and of his family, including food, clothing, housing and medical care and necessary social services, and the right to security in the event of unemployment, sickness, disability, widowhood, old age or other lack of livelihood in circumstances beyond his control. [9]

This is a political statement of goals, because it doesn't indicate how these rights will be achieved. However, the fact that they exist, on paper, agreed to by almost all of the members of the UN at the time and regularly re-affirmed, provides a touchstone for programs and processes aimed at achieving them. There is also a comparable statement regarding the relationship of social justice to health, health care, and medicine. In 1978, the World Health Organization (WHO) issued the "Declaration of Alma-Ata" at a conference held in that city (now called Almaty, it was then but is no longer the capital of Kazakhstan). It defined "health" as "...a state of complete physical, mental and social wellbeing, and not merely the absence of disease or infirmity..." and asserted that it "... is a fundamental human right... "

This has been an important cornerstone statement for the development of health care and primary care for more than 40 years. Primary Health Care, which was also defined at Alma-Ata, is integrally tied to the definition of health:

Primary health care is essential health care based on practical, scientifically sound and socially acceptable methods and technology made universally accessible to individuals and families in the community through their full participation and at a cost that the community and country can afford to maintain at every stage of their development in the spirit of self-reliance and self-determination.

In these definitions, healthcare is not limited to medical care, and it is, again as a goal, called on to be "universally" accessible. However, this statement also accounts for the varying economic ability of different countries. I once heard a presentation on the Mexican healthcare system, which described a structure to provide universally accessible care, but it did not always achieve this goal. I concluded that in Mexico, they have the *desire* to provide universal access, but not the resources, while in the U.S. we have the *resources* but not the desire. This is far less defensible.

Many countries, richer than Mexico, have developed a functional universal health system; indeed all countries in the Organization for Economic Cooperation and Development (OECD) have, except for the United States. Our closest neighbor, Canada, has a universal health system based on a single payer (the government) but relying mainly on private physicians. Canadian Medicare (that is the name of their program), actually 13 systems run by each province, is held together by five principles: they must be *publicly administered, comprehensive, universal, portable* (i.e., residents of one province must be covered in other provinces), and *accessible*. It is not perfect, certainly, but it is highly valued by Canadians. In 2004, the Canadian Broadcasting System ran a special program called "The Greatest Canadian." After extensive polling, the top 10 vote-getters were read in alphabetical order, and a celebrity argued the case for each. In the second round of polling the 10 were voted on again. Some of the names are familiar to Americans, including Alexander Graham Bell (#9) and Wayne Gretzky (#10). But the winner, the person determined to be the Greatest Canadian, probably isn't a familiar name to Americans—Tommy Douglas, the father of the Canadian health system. That Canada's health system is so highly valued by Canadians, whatever its problems may be, that the force behind bringing it into being is seen as the greatest Canadian is, I think, a very impressive testimony to that program.

As has become clear, values underpin and guide the values of this book. Proponents of other health care system (such as the current one in the U.S.) have other values, and it's imperative to understand where advocates for different systems are coming from. I do not think that it is possible to decide what to do, what direction to head in, what strategy to use, what system to develop, without knowing where we want to go, and it is our values that inform this. While we may agree on a set of values, or a particular goal, it is all too common for people and institutions, from organizations to governments, to movements, to get so immersed in the details of implementing a program that it can lose sight of the reason it is engaged in its effort. I unequivocally come down on the side of justice as a value, of a more healthy society as a value, of systems, programs, and interventions that enhance health rather than profit as a value.

Do we want to achieve a better world, one in which people are more healthy, one in which the things that we know how to do to increase health are available to everyone, to move from potential to achievable for the entire population? Do we want to create a more just world, one which eliminates inequities and decreases inequalities? If we do, we must ensure that we raise our heads out of the weeds, and go beyond continuing to do what we know how to do. If we are to design a new system to achieve goals that are different from those the current system is designed for we must make sure that we know what these goals are, what the basic reasons we are doing our work are, what our values are.

We are not born equal, and if we are to have equity we need to take that into account. As we develop new systems and new strategies, we must keep in mind the goals that we are trying to achieve, the values that motivate us. If we just *do* things, even things we have decided in the past were wise, without reflecting on their impact, we risk becoming technocrats who get lost in the process of change and may forget to raise our heads from our work for long enough to be sure that we are still headed in the direction we want to go.

History is often seen to be the ultimate judge of whether a strategy was successful (certainly recognizing Tommy Douglas as the "Greatest Canadian" is an example), but values must be the yardstick against which we measure success. Different strategies will be "successful" if we seek a more equal, more just society than if we want one that is less equal (and, to be sure, there are those who do).

I believe that health care is a basic right, a human right, as identified by the Universal Declaration of Human Rights. Journalist T.R. Reid visited 5 capitalist countries (the UK, Japan, Germany, Switzerland, and Taiwan) for his PBS special *Sick Around the World*.[10] Given that medical care is the single largest cause of personal bankruptcy in the U.S.,[11] one of the questions that he asked leaders in each country was how many of their citizens went bankrupt as a result of health care debts. They all answered "none." The most dramatic response was from the President of the Swiss Confederation, a conservative who had originally opposed the Swiss program in the early 1990s. "*No one,*" he boomed in his French- accented English, "*why, it would be a national scandal!*"

Indeed it should be, because the health of our society depends upon the health of all of us.

When people crowd our emergency rooms, not with minor illnesses, but with serious illnesses that could have been prevented with earlier treatment, that is a scandal.

When parents cannot afford their own health care and their

illnesses threaten their ability to keep providing for their children, that is a scandal.

When people stay in jobs they hate, or forego the opportunity to start a new business, because they rightfully fear being uninsured, that is a scandal.

When our friends and neighbors, parents and children, only take partial doses of their medicine because it is a choice between that and not eating, that is a scandal.

When a hard-working man with chest pain can see the billboards advertising the superb heart care available at our local hospitals and know they are not meant for him because he is uninsured, that is a scandal.

We need to understand how our system is broken, what it is focused on and what we must do to fix that system or build a new one and focus it on providing health care that strengthens everyone in the country. To understand how the system is broken, I will look at some data on the social determinants of health (housing, food, education, safety, etc.) and their impact upon our society, in particular health disparities. I will then look at what the required components of a good health care system are in the next chapter, specifically the benefits that accrue to a health system from primary care and its centrality, both for the functional system and for the benefit of the health of both populations and individuals. I will emphasize the importance of keeping our focus on people, not diseases. I will then look at medical education, and to some degree health professions education in general, in the U.S., and how its structure and content contribute to the current dysfunctional system and how changes to it might help lead us in the right direction.

The next question is about medicine itself, how it functions to provide care and how it, and science, is often misunderstood by the public, and why. In this section I will address medical communication, between health professionals and their patients. Another crucial aspect of that communication is how media coverage shapes patient expectations, and how it can both clarify and obscure the applied science of healthcare. This leads directly to the role of profit and the ways in which it impacts, and in my opinion usually perverts, the healthcare system, driving demand for products and services among both providers and patients, encouraging the pursuit of certain profitable "product lines" by healthcare providers, and creating an incentive that is different from, and often in conflict with, the health of people.

Having outlined the problems, my final section will examine proposed solutions, and their likely outcomes. I will draw on the information presented in the earlier chapters, and in particular on the concepts examined here, on keeping our eyes on the prize, on achieving the highest level of health possible for our population and the individuals people who comprise it. Much discussion in the last few years has focused on achieving the "triple aim" of healthcare: (improved) quality, (greater) patient satisfaction, and (lower) cost. To this I would add (enhanced) access, because without access there cannot be quality. As pointed out by Schiff, Bindman, and Brennan, denial of care is the "gravest of all quality defects."[12] All of these, however, are about the medical care system rather than the social determinants of health. It will be critical to identify not just where and how money can be saved, but where and how money can be used most effectively to enhance people's health.

I do think we need to go upstream and see what is happening, and try to intervene and prevent bad outcomes. In medical care, and in healthcare in general, we are continuously refining our technology, getting better and faster (and more expensive), but we often do not look to causes. And when we find causes that are beyond our ability to intervene on and change, like social injustice, poverty, lack of access to food and housing and education and jobs, and hope, we throw up our hands and, essentially say "more technology!" We need to internalize a broader understanding of the determinants of health, as illustrated in the model from *Healthy People 2010* (see page 50), but we also need to broaden our conception of what medicine and health care can do.

The case is solid for the claim that our system is broken and we need to focus on different values, and I will present data in this book to support my opinions and conclusions. As discussed above, it is only by identifying our values and keeping them in mind and in sight that we can evaluate whether what we are doing is good and taking us in the right direction.

When we are all in it together, we all have an interest in making the system be as good as it can be. The efforts of those of us who are more educated, more financially able, more vocal, more empowered will ensure that the needs of those who are less able to lobby for themselves are also met. Just as our nation cannot survive half-slave and half-free, or with only half of adults having the vote, we cannot survive with only some of us having access to health care.

We need to do this for all of us, for ultimately, after all, we are indeed our brothers' and sisters' keepers.

References

1. http://www.dartmouth.edu/~cecs/hcild/hcild.html
2. National Research Council and Institute of Medicine. U.S. Health in International Perspective: Shorter Lives, Poorer Health. Washington, DC: The National Academies Press, 2013. http://www.iom.edu/Reports/2013/US-Health-in-International-Perspective-Shorter-Lives-Poorer-Health.aspx
3. Woolf, S., The U.S. Health Disadvantage, plenary presentation at Society of Teachers of Family Medicine Annual Conference, May, 2014, San Antonio TX. Available at http://www.fmdrl.org.
4. Farmer P, How we can save millions of lives, *New York Times*, November 17, 2011. http://www.washingtonpost.com/opinions/how-we-can-save-millions-of-lives/2011/11/11/gIQAf1rBWN_story.html
5. Belmont report, Ethical Principles for Research involving Human Subjects, Federal Register V. 44 No. 76 p. 23192, April 18, 1979. https://web.archive.org/web/20111017133845/http://www.hhs.gov/ohrp/archive/documents/19790418.pdf
6. Kirch DG, Vernon DJ, The ethical foundation of American medicine: in search of social justice, *JAMA*; 301(14):1482-4, Apr.8,2009
7. Rawls J. A *Theory of Justice*. Belknap Press. Cambridge MA. 1971. p. 303.
8. Inscribed on a plaque at the FDR Memorial, Washington, DC.
9. United Nations, The Universal Declaration of Human Rights, http://www.un.org/en/documents/udhr/index.shtml
10. Reid TR, PBS Frontline: Sick around the world. http://www.pbs.org/wgbh/pages/frontline/sickaroundtheworld/
11. Mangan D, Medical Bills Are the Biggest Cause of US Bankruptcies: Study, CNBC, June 25, 2013. http://www.cnbc.com/id/100840148#.
12. Schiff GD, Bindman AB, Brennan TA,. A better-quality alternative: Single-payer national health system reform. Physicians for a National Health Program Quality of Care Working Group. *JAMA*. 272(10):803-8, Sept 14, 1994

Chapter 2

The U.S. Healthcare System:
Best in the World?

The United States today devotes 16 percent of its gross do-
mestic product to medical care, more per capita than any
other nation in the world. Yet numerous measures indicate
the country lags in overall health: It ranks 29th in infant
mortality, 48th in life expectancy and 19th out of 19 indus-
trialized nations in preventable deaths.[1]

—Commonwealth Fund

We often hear, from politicians and television talking heads who are opposing major change in the way healthcare is covered and provided in the United States that "we have the best health-care system in the world." Overall the data show that we do not. "We have the best medical care in the world" may be a little closer to the truth, but only for those who are lucky and relatively well-to-do, and even they often get care that they do not need and may put them at risk.

What is true is that, in the U.S., the most difficult, demanding, and dramatic care can be obtained, provided one has the money to pay for it. This is why billionaire oil sheiks come to this country for their surgery and for what Donald Berwick calls "rescue care." If you need high-tech, highly-complex treatments, U.S. hospitals can offer the best in the world, if you have the money or the insurance coverage. The irony is that if you do, you may find yourself getting high-tech, highly complex treatments even when you don't really need them, while if you don't have the money, they may be unavailable to you even when they would be of great benefit. However, as the data I cite in the opening chapter demonstrate, the overall effect of our healthcare system is, in the title of the report from the Institute of Medicine report *Shorter Lives, Poorer Health*.[2] Our significant health indicators, such as life expectancy and infant mortality, lag behind those of other wealthy countries and many that are not so wealthy. That we have the most costly healthcare system, however, is not open to debate.

What data provide a picture of the overall health of Americans or compares it to that of other countries? The data have been starkly consistent for many years, and demonstrate that the main thing that U.S. health care leads the world in is cost, not in health outcomes. Many expressed shock when, in 2000, the World Health Organization (WHO) released *The World Health Report 2000 - Health Systems: Improving Performance*.[3] While relative to all countries the U.S. was far from the bottom (because there are so many poor countries), it ranked 37th in the world, behind all wealthy other industrialized western nations; it was just behind Costa Rica and just ahead of Slovenia.

These data are now quite old, and the WHO has not released a more recent version of the report, so have things changed significantly in this time? No. Many other international comparisons have been done, and their results are consistent. The Commonwealth Fund produces one of the most thorough sets of studies, issuing reports comparing the U.S. health status to other nations. Its 2008 report, *Why Not The Best?*, establishes health-system benchmarks based on performance in the best-performing nations in 5 dimensions: Healthy Lives, Quality, Access, Efficiency, and Equity, as well as an Overall score. With the benchmark set as 100, the U.S. overall score was 65, down from 67 in the report from 2006. In the individual areas, the U.S. score was slightly up in Equity (70 to 71) and in Efficiency (52 to 53—but this remained the lowest-performing dimension), and was down in all the other dimensions, including Healthy Lives. To achieve this performance the U.S. was at the time spending 16% of its gross domestic product on health care, nearly twice that of the other developed nations on a per capita basis.[4] The *Washington Post* noted that:

> *The United States today devotes 16 percent of its gross domestic product to medical care, more per capita than any other nation in the world. Yet numerous measures indicate the country lags in overall health: It ranks 29th in infant mortality, 48th in life expectancy and 19th out of 19 industrialized nations in preventable deaths.[5]*

In 2010 and again in 2014, the Commonwealth Fund's updated its report, *Mirror, Mirror on the Wall.*[6] Did things get better for the U.S.? No. The latest report compares 11 industrialized countries. The higher the score, the lower the ranking and the worse a country is doing. The U.S. total for the 5 main dimensions of health care (Quality, Access, Efficiency, Equity, and Healthy Lives) was 47, ranking #11 out of 11. It did this while spending $8,508 per capita, by far the most of any of the countries. The best rank was the UK with a score of 15; it also spent the second least, $3,405 per capita (40% of U.S. per capita spending). The U.S. also ranked #11 in 3 of the 5 dimensions measured (Efficiency, Equity and Healthy Lives), and its highest rank was #5 (Quality). The UK, by contrast, was #1 in all dimensions except Equity (#2), and Healthy Lives (#10, ahead of only the U.S.). Interestingly, the Netherlands, which was #1 of the 7 countries evaluated in the 2010 report (France, Norway, Sweden, and Switzerland were added for 2014) dropped to #5. This has coincided with a highly-publicized move of the Dutch health system to a more "market based" approach.[7] Figure 2.1 reproduces the Commonwealth Fund table; Figure 2.2 presents the total score on the five dimensions versus the per capita expenditure of these 11 countries.

Figure 2.1

Overall Ranking of Eleven Health Care Systems

COUNTRY RANKINGS
Top 2*
Middle
Bottom 2*

	AUS	CAN	FRA	GER	NETH	NZ	NOR	SWE	SWIZ	UK	US
OVERALL RANKING (2013)	4	10	9	5	5	7	7	3	2	1	11
Quality Care	2	9	8	7	5	4	11	10	3	1	5
Effective Care	4	7	9	6	5	2	11	10	8	1	3
Safe Care	3	10	2	6	7	9	11	5	4	1	7
Coordinated Care	4	8	9	10	5	2	7	11	3	1	6
Patient-Centered Care	5	8	10	7	3	6	11	9	2	1	4
Access	8	9	11	2	4	7	6	4	2	1	9
Cost-Related Problem	9	5	10	4	8	6	3	1	7	1	11
Timeliness of Care	6	11	10	4	2	7	8	9	1	3	5
Efficiency	4	10	8	9	7	3	4	2	6	1	11
Equity	5	9	7	4	8	10	6	1	2	2	11
Healthy Lives	4	8	1	7	5	9	6	2	3	10	11
Health Expenditures/Capita, 2011**	$3,800	$4,522	$4,118	$4,495	$5,099	$3,182	$5,669	$3,925	$5,643	$3,405	$8,508

Notes: *Includes ties, **Expenditures shown in $US PPP (Purchasing Power Parity). Australian $ data from 2010.

Source: Reprinted with permission from Davis, K, Stremikis, K, Squires, D et al. *Mirror, Mirror on the Wall, 2014 Update: How the U.S. Health Care System Compares Internationally.* The Commonwealth Fund, June 16, 2014.

Figure 2.2

Health System Score vs. Cost

Commonwealth Fund, 2014

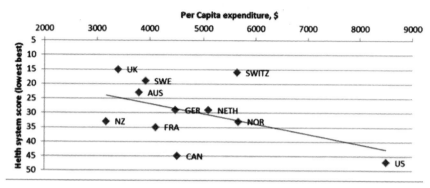

source: Reprinted with permission of the Commonwealth Fund

Of the 10 countries to which the U.S. is compared, 7 are in Europe (France, Germany, the Netherlands, Norway, Sweden, Switzerland and the United Kingdom), but the health status of Americans is below that of most European countries, increasingly including those from the former Eastern bloc, such as Slovenia. And, in addition to having overall poorer health status, the difference in health status between rich and poor is greater in the U.S. than in European countries. In a comparison of 16 wealthy countries in terms of mortality amenable to health care (deaths that could have been prevented by health care), in the 10 years from 1997 to 2007 the U.S. improved (from 120 to 96 per 100,000) but other countries improved more, so that in the later estimate it has moved from 14th to last of the 16 comparison countries (Figure 2.3).[8]

To understand these issues, a group of researchers examined overall health status and the impact of wealth on health, in the

Figure 2.3

U.S. Lags Other Countries: Mortality Amenable to Health Care

Deaths per 100,000 population

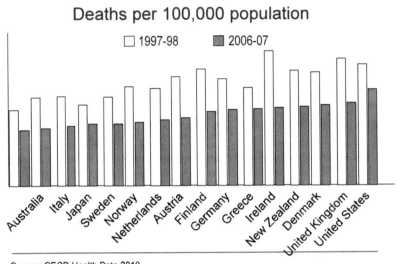

Source: OECD Health Data 2010

U.S. and in Europe. The goal of the study was to look at the health differences that exist between Americans and Europeans and assess whether wealth is a factor in those differences, and whether there are differences in Europe as well. In other words, it looked at both the difference in health between wealthy and poor Americans and wealthy and poor Europeans (comparing "tertiles", top, middle and bottom thirds of wealth within each country, to minimize the impact of differences in wealth between countries) as well as the overall difference between Americans and Europeans, looking separately at the UK and considering the rest of Europe together.

The study examined 9,900 Americans aged 50-74 and compared them to 6,500 British and 17,000 mainland Europeans in the same age range. To exclude the effect of racial disparities only non-Latino white U.S. adults were included in the study. The results were consistent with other work demonstrating the relatively poor health status of the U.S.:

The rate for every disease examined was higher in the U.S. adults than in either the English or European groups. Rates of cancer in the U.S. were 11%, while they were 6% in England and 5% in Europe. Heart disease rates were 18% in the U.S., 12% in Britain, and 11% in Europe.

In all groups the rate of disease was higher in the poorer than in the wealthier groups, except for cancer, which is apparently an equal-opportunity disease.

The difference between rich and poor was much greater in the U.S. and England than in Europe.[9] While the poorest Britons had over twice the odds of having heart disease as the richest, slightly more than in the U.S., the overall rate of heart disease was only 2/3 of that in the U.S. (12% vs 18% repectively). Thus, all British groups are doing significantly better than their U.S. counterparts.[10]

Within the U.S., health status varies among different segments of the population. These differences, or disparities, are more properly described as inequities when they result from conditions that could be changed (as opposed to differences that cannot be addressed with current knowledge, such as those based on age and genetics). The differences have been examined in terms of wealth (or class or socioeconomic status), as in the previous study, in terms of race/ethnicity, and in terms of geographic location. It turns out that there are in fact differences in the health status of Americans between different regions and states. These differences reflect in part differences in wealth and racial/ethnic composition in these states and regions, but most importantly a state's approach to health and social services for its residents, particularly those with the greatest need. While these policies are carried out at the state level, states in the same region often have similar policies, resulting in differences that can be seen at the regional level.

The Commonwealth Fund 2013 scorecard, *Health Care in the Two Americas,* sought to identify these differences.[11] They discovered very large differences in the health status and health care received by the low income populations in "high-performing" and "low-performing" states, with much less difference in health status among high-income people living in different states. To put that another way, wealthier people did about the same no matter where they lived, while poor people did much worse in certain states. There was a definite regionalization, with the highest performing states clustered in the Northeast and North Central regions and Hawaii, and the lowest performing states in the South and South Central regions (Figure 2.4).

These differences reflect the degree to which states (and state groups) choose to expend resources on health care and on the social services that play a major role in determining health. However, no state is in the top quartile in all 30 of the Commonwealth Fund's measures, although some are in the bottom quartile in virtually all measures. Poverty is clearly associated with poor health status, as will be further discussed in Chapter 4, but some states and regions do more to mitigate these effects than others. Overall, the U.S. has worse health status, for both its poor and its overall population, than do European countries. The fact is that within the U.S. those states and regions that provide more support for people, ensure that they have housing, food and education as well as financial ac-

Figure 2.4

Overall Health Performance
For Low-Income Populations

Deaths per 100,000 population

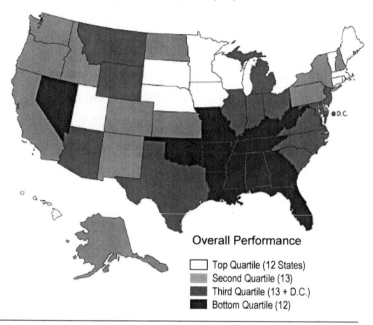

Overall Performance

☐ Top Quartile (12 States)
▨ Second Quartile (13)
▧ Third Quartile (13 + D.C.)
■ Bottom Quartile (12)

Source: The Commonwealth Fund. Reprinted with permission. Available at http://www.
commonwealthfund.org/publications/fund-reports/2013/sep/low-income-scorecard

cess to health care, and have a strong primary care infrastructure, move them further from the edge of the cliff (see p. 45), have a fence that keeps them from falling off as easily, and provide a safety net to decrease the likelihood that they will find themselves crashing to the ground below, have far better health status. In the U.S., we have a well-developed structure for picking up the bodies and repairing those that can be repaired (and even intervening when the benefit is little, or interventions can be harmful), but this does little to maintain the health of the population.

Shouldering Costs:
The Conundrum Faced by Every System

Every country faces a simple problem: sick people use the most health care and cost the most, while healthy people cost next to nothing. If only sick people pay for care, they can't shoulder the burden of treatment for expensive conditions such as cancer, catastrophic injuries and chronic diseases. The question every society faces is, how do you spread that cost widely enough so that people who need the care don't hesitate to use it for fear of financial ruin, and once they get that care aren't shattered by the costs? Continuing our comparison of the U.S. and other countries, we look at two broad answers: a single payer system where that cost is shouldered by the government (and spread across the taxpayers), and private insurance, which is paid for by people buying a range of policies.

We save the question "which system delivers the best health outcomes?" for later. Here we are focused on how the U.S. is approaching the issue. Having examined data on overall health status in the U.S. compared to other developed countries, on the differences in health within U.S. states and regions, as well as the degree to which health status is related to poverty and other social factors, it is clear that the U.S. lags behind its counterparts in the developed world.

Although poor people, racial and ethnic minorities, and those who live in geographically remote areas, are more likely to be sick than those who are more well off, are white, or live in urban settings, there are sick people from all of these groups. And it is sick people who cost money to care for, regardless of the way that system is organized or paid for. The way that the system is organized and paid for does matter in the overall cost, however, which is why costs are so high in the U.S..

Many Americans misunderstand how health care costs work. Simply, most of the money is not spent on most of the people. While there have been excellent journalistic reports about health costs (notably those of Elisabeth Rosenthal in the *New York Times*), many journalists who write episodically about health care are living in middle-class, young-to-middle aged worlds, and are among the worst perpetrators of misunderstanding healthcare usage. The stories they write often are about their rotator cuff surgery or their neighbor's strep throat. In fact, however, about 50% of the population accounts for only 3% of health care costs; thus half of us are essentially "rounding error." At the other end of the spectrum, about 5% of people account for 50% of costs. The remainder are using about "their share" of health dollars as depicted in Figure 2.5.

That is, if $100 were spent on 100 people (whose costs are distributed as per the whole population), 45 people would cost about "their share", about $1 each, 50 people would cost $0.06 (6 cents) each, and 5 people would cost $10 each.

The "mid-users" who are using about "their share" are those who have chronic health problems and have to go to doctors more frequently, and get more tests, but don't have frequent hospitalizations. It also includes the folks who in most years are in the low-use group but, in a given year, have surgery or physical therapy—like for those rotator cuffs. This part of the population includes a disproportionate percent of seniors, who have more chronic disease and use more health care services.

Because seniors are also more likely to have multiple chron-

Figure 2.5

Percent of Population

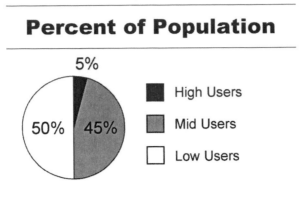

5%

50% 45%

High Users

Mid Users

Low Users

Percent of
Health Care Costs

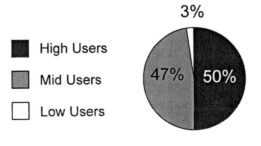

High Users

Mid Users

Low Users

3%

47% 50%

ic health problems that require multiple hospitalizations, and because they are more likely to have cancer, which costs a lot to treat, they are also disproportionately represented in the high user group. However, they are still the minority of that group. These high-cost users also include other people with cancer, people with major trauma (such as from auto accidents) requiring multiple surgeries, and premature and sick babies requiring extremely expensive care in neonatal intensive care units.

This lopsided usage by a small number of people is a very important concept: it is the reason that insurance companies historically have "cherry picked" healthy patients, and why one of the main parts of the Affordable Care Act (ACA) is that people cannot be denied coverage because of pre-existing conditions. It is also why, for good reason, the insurance companies insisted upon the "individual mandate", because if everyone were not required to buy insurance those who were healthy would wait until they were sick before they bought health insurance. This is the basic concept of insurance—lots of people pay in but only some people "benefit." I put "benefit" in quotation marks because for almost all types of insurance, it requires something bad to happen to "benefit": having a car accident (for auto insurance), being robbed or having your house burn down (for homeowners insurance), dying (for life insurance), or getting sick (for health insurance).

The problem with the remedy proposed for insurance company "cherry picking" is that, given the above data, insurers don't have to enroll only people in the "low cost" group (although I'm sure they'd like that); they just have to find subtle ways to get rid of one or two of those 5 high-cost people. For each one of those people they can avoid insuring, they save the same amount as their cost for 10 "mid-user" people or 167 "low users." For the ACA to work as expected, each insurance company would have to enroll 5% of the high users, but this is impossible in large part because we don't always know who they're going to be in the future; this is also why insurers cannot be sure that they have none of them.

So if everyone looks at it from the point of view of their current self-interest, those in that "low use, low cost" group wouldn't want to pay more for all those high-cost, high-use folks. This year, today, it wouldn't be in our self-interest. Except that we don't know when we, or our teenage children, will be in a car accident that rockets them from the low-cost to the high-cost group. And we don't know when we'll have a premature baby, or be diagnosed with cancer. Or have us, or our parents, move from the mid-cost, have-chronic-conditions-and-see-the-doctor-but-rarely-be-hospitalized group to the "red" high-cost be-hospitalized-a-lot- including-in-intensive-care group.

The result is that we are all in it together. It makes sense to solve the issues of "cherry picking" and excessive risk, as well as the enormous cost involved in insurance company profit, by having only one system, one insurance plan in which everyone is covered, such as the single-payer system in Canada. Or, as a slightly more complex alternative, a single-benefit system as in Switzerland, where there are multiple payers (insurance companies) but they all must provide the same core benefits and are non-profit, so they must compete on service, not price. Having a system that includes *everyone,* even those left out by the ACA (whether that system more resembles Canada or Switzerland or another country) will not be sufficient to guarantee that Americans would have the same health benefit as other wealthy nations because there are still the social determinants of health. However, even though it is not sufficient, it is necessary.

Every other country with the resources to provide for the health and the health care of its people has done a better job of it than we have.

A comparison of health care systems is illuminating, but we are actually getting ahead of ourselves. The greatest impacts on public health actually have to do with what happens to people *before* they get sick: Do they have running water? Do they get enough good food to eat (and not too much bad food)? What are their job prospects and education like? We turn to this discussion next.

References

1. Davis, K., Stremikis, K., Squires D. et al. *Mirror, Mirror on the Wall, 2014 update,* How the U.S. Health Care System Compares Internationally. Commonwealth Fund, June 16, 2014.

2. National Research Council and Institute of Medicine. U.S. Health in International Perspective: Shorter Lives, Poorer Health. Washington, DC: The National Academies Press, 2013. http://www.iom.edu/Reports/2013/US-Health-in-International-Perspective-Shorter-Lives-Poorer-Health.aspx

3. World Health Organization, *The world health report 2000 - Health systems: improving performance,* Geneva, 2000. http://www.who.int/whr/2000/en/index.html.

4. *The Commonwealth Fund Commission on a High Performance Health System, Why Not the Best? Results from the National Scorecard on U.S. Health System Performance, 2008,* The Commonwealth Fund, July 2008., http://www.commonwealthfund.org/Publications/Fund-Reports/2008/Jul/Why-Not-the-Best—Results-from-the-National-Scorecard-on-U-S—Health-System-Performance—2008.aspx

5. Ibid #1.

6. Davis, K, Stremikis, K, Squires, D, et all, *Mirror, Mirror on the Wall: How the Performance of the U.S. Health Care System Compares Internationally, 2014 Update,* The Commonwealth Fund, June 2014. http://www.commonwealthfund.org/publications/fund-reports/2014/jun/mirror-mirror

7. Schäfer W, et al., The Netherlands Health System Review, *Health Systems in Transition,* Vol 12, No 1, 2010.

8. Commonwealth Fund, U.S. Ranks Last Among High-Income Nations on Preventable Deaths, Lagging Behind as Others Improve More Rapidly, http://www.commonwealthfund.org/publications/press-releases/2011/sep/us-ranks-last-on-preventable-deaths

9. Avedano M, MM Glymour, J Banks, J Mackenbach, Health disadvantage in U.S. adults aged 50 to 74 years: A comparison of the health of rich and poor Americans with that of Europeans, *Am J Pub Health* 99(3):540, Mar 2009

10. Ibid # 9

11. Schoen,C., Radley, D. C., Riley,P., et all, *Health Care in the Two Americas: Findings from the Scorecard on State Health System Performance for Low-Income Populations, 2013.* The Commonwealth Fund, September 2013. http://www.commonwealthfund.org/Publications/Fund-Reports/2013/Sep/Low-Income-Scorecard.aspx

Chapter 3

The Social Determinants
of Health and Health Inequities

*The availability of health care is inversely proportional to
the need for it.*

—Julian Tudor Hart[1]

In 1848, the Prussian government sent a young physician
named Rudolf Virchow to investigate an outbreak of typhus in the
coal-mining region of Upper Silesia. He concluded that the main
cause of the typhus outbreak was the social and economic situation of the residents of the region. Although Virchow later became famous for advancing cell theory, and his name is attached
to dozens of medical eponyms (Virchow's node, Virchow cells,
Virchow's autopsy, etc.), he may be best known as the "Father of
Social Medicine." His 1848 report is one of the first clear discussions of the social determinants of health, the realization that it is
the circumstances of people's lives, their socioeconomic status,
the housing they live in, the food they eat, the environmental ex-
posures they have, their ability to access basic needs in the best
of times and the margin of safety that they have when times grow
more difficult, that are most important in health and disease.[2]

Of course, today we see much less typhus, at least in the U.S.,
but we still see much disease that results from social conditions.
In Gregory Nava's 1983 film *El Norte*,[3] one of the lead characters

actually dies from typhus. She has finally reached Los Angeles after a long and grueling journey from Guatemala, but succumbs to the disease contracted when she was crawling through sewers trying to get into this country. If we ask "Why did she get typhus?" the "medical" answer would be that she was bitten by a rat-flea carrying the pathogenic organism *Rickettsia typhae*. But this answer is inadequate: she would likely not have contracted the disease if she had not been crawling through sewers. The next question must be "Why was she crawling through a sewer?" Finally, our most important social question must be "What is wrong with a situation in which a person finds that crawling through a sewer infested with rats, fleas, and *Rickettsia typhae* is a risk worth taking?"

The "social determinants of health" are a key component of social justice. To the extent that our social circumstances create health disparities, more properly called inequities because they are not just differences but differences that are both to the disadvantage of a portion of the population and are remediable, they reflect a less-than-just society. More than a century after Virchow, the British physician Julian Tudor Hart, the sole doctor practicing in the Welsh coal-mining town of Glyncorrwg in the middle of the twentieth century, was able to identify who got sick from what and how it related to their economic and social standing. As an epidemiologist he gathered these data (in the pre-computer era), and then expanded them by looking at access to health care across Britain. The result was a 1971 article in *Lancet* called "The Inverse Care Law", in which he demonstrated with empiric data that "the availability of health care services is inversely proportional to the need for it."[4]

The work of Tudor Hart, Virchow, and many since then, has demonstrated that it is more than the availability of health services that are inversely proportional to the need for them. It is to a larger and more significant extent the availability of the opportunity to be healthy. This means having an income sufficient to ensure adequate housing and food, to have heat in the winter, to have neighborhoods that are safe enough to be active in without risking your life, to have parks and sidewalks. It means having communities in which healthful food is available at a price that you can afford. It means having jobs that do not make you sick, and that pay you enough that you don't need to have two or three to get by and thus have time for healthful living. It means having communities where people support each other, where the stress of just getting by isn't enough to overwhelm you.

Social determinants of health may well be more important than health care itself. But although this may be true, it begs the question: are they treatable? Can a doctor or other health care provider actually do anything about these age-old problems? This chapter sets out first to understand what these social determinants are and then to answer that question. Changing the social determinants is a big task, beyond that of any individual, even an individual health care worker, but not beyond the capability of society as a whole. Understanding how they work will help us shape a health care system that takes them into account, that seeks to provide the best health care possible in contexts where we have to battle against those determinants, and work to change them. We will now look at how providers can do this more.

In the 1960s, Michael Marmot and his colleagues at the University of London began an examination into the relationship of social status to health, now known collectively as the Whitehall Studies. They sought to discover the influence of social class on health by looking at British civil servants in Whitehall, the seat of government. This was important, because it controlled for differences in the characteristics of the workplace such as exposure to industrial toxins, higher physical risk for factory workers and outdoor workers, and any other such difference that might be the result of the place that they worked; these people worked in the same offices. They also controlled for known risk factors such as smoking that might have been more prevalent in one class than another. They discovered that health, and mortality, are highly linked to class, and that there is a linear increase in life expectancy and health status with increasing class. The later Whitehall II studies in the 1980s began to elucidate many of the characteristics that might lead to these outcomes, including the stress of survival.[5] Simply put, the stress of having to decide whether to pay the rent or feed your children is of a different order than whether to have your skiing vacation in St. Moritz or Gstaad. This degree of stress has a significant negative impact on your health, through at least two paths. One is through neuroendocrine mechanisms that result in high levels of "stress" hormones such as cortisol that have a direct physical effect on the body (good in short-term crises, bad over the long haul). The other is that when your time and money are used up with just trying to get by, there is much less of both for healthful eating, exercise, and relaxation.

The greatest determinants of health of populations are those that come before medical care, even before primary care, which will be the subject of Chapter 5. The extent to which a society lacks social justice is reflected in differences in social determinants, which have a proportionally greater impact upon the health of the population and the production of health disparities. This is simply and clearly demonstrated in the "cliff analogy", developed by Camara Phyllis Jones and colleagues. (Figure 3.1).[6] They graphically demonstrate that, while all people are at risk for injury or illness, some live a little—or a lot—closer to the "edge," which puts them at greater risk of falling off, i.e., developing illness or injury. The same is obviously true for populations who live "closer to the edge", who are at higher risk for disease—because of genetic risks, environmental risks, and behavioral risks—but also because they have less money, or social support, or greater stress in their lives.[7] Things that, at the best of times, mean they are just able to get by and keep from falling off.

Figure 3.1

Cliff Analogy to the
Social Determinants of Health

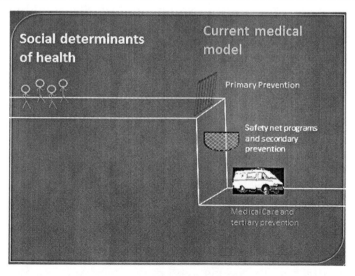

Source: graphic reprinted with permission from Neil Palafax, M.D., based upon Jones, CP, Jones, CY, Perry, GS. Addressing the social determinants of children's health: A cliff analogy. *J Health Care for the Poor and Underserved*, 20 (4): 1-12, 2009.

Jones' cliff analogy goes on further to look at what we can do:

- We can pick up the person, or people, who "fall off the cliff", who get sick. This is known as "tertiary prevention", because the bad thing has already happened and we are hoping to prevent complications, prevent it from getting worse. This is where we spend almost all of our "healthcare" dollars.

- Or maybe we can put up a safety net. "Safety net clinics" and "safety net hospitals" can be thought of as a form of secondary prevention—people have already "fallen", their high blood pressure or diabetes has become uncontrolled and they are at risk for something really bad. So—we intervene.

- Or we could actually put a fence up on the edge of the cliff, preventing people from falling off. This is a kind of "primary prevention", like vaccinations, and cancer screening, and education about healthful behaviors.

All these activities, done at the "cliff face", are components of medical care. But there is something else that might be even more effective: moving these people further from the edge. That way, when they need health care, things won't be quite so precarious. This "pre-primary" prevention actually involves intervening on the core risk factors for health—addressing the social determinants of health. Much to our society's detriment, we do not emphasize addressing them, focusing instead on an almost entirely medical model.

This is what health inequities are about. They are about differences that do not have to be there, about people who are at greater risk because they have poorer food or housing, who live in dangerous neighborhoods, who may not have adequate access to preventive and primary care, may not have safety-net services, and may not even have the ambulance come as quickly. Inequities are about differences that do not have to be present. Poor people are always at greater risk, but as discussed in Chapter 2, many other countries have done a much better job of addressing these social determinants as well as improving access to medical care.

If we fix the problem of access to medical care, as ACA has just begun to do, not addressing the social determinants will continue to leave people in poorer health. This fact is often ignored, dismissed, or is simply outside the ken of many people, including many who should know better, because sometimes it is simply convenient to ignore it. For example, the ACA contains a "pay for performance" section that financially rewards hospitals for meeting certain standards of quality of care. This is good, but some have expressed concern that these payments are not adjusted for the neediness of the patient population cared for by the hospital, thus effectively rewarding hospitals who care for the most well-to-do and penalizing those who care for the poorest.[8] The flaw is that it ignores the social determinants of health, because it implies that a hospital can get the same outcomes caring for the poorest, least educated, and most poorly housed as in caring for the most privileged.

The justification for this policy, as put forward by the director of quality measurement programs at the federal Centers for Medicare and Medicaid Services (CMS), which runs Medicare, is that:

"We do not want to hold hospitals to different standards of care simply because they treat a large number of low-socio-economic-status patients. Our position has always been not to risk-adjust for socioeconomic status within our measures

because of concern about masking disparities, and poten-
tially rewarding providers who provide a lower level of care
for minorities or poor patients."[9]

This sounds noble, and indeed, the concept of justice requires that all people receive the same level of care, that they have the same options for treatment, and that different quality of care is not provided to those with greater resources. However, the argument made by CMS chooses to ignore those other factors—the social determinants of health—that precede accessing the health care system and largely determine what will happen after discharge. For example, holding a hospital financially responsible if a patient is readmitted without taking to account the different circumstances into which people are discharged is unreasonable. Going home to a clean environment with people to care for you and an opportunity to rest and eat healthful food is different from going home to a poorly-heated, drafty place where you live alone and cannot afford food or medication—or to no home at all. Obviously, it would be best if those social conditions could be fixed, rather than "controlled for", but if they are not, it is disingenuous to ignore how they impact medical outcomes.

Personal Responsibility, Victim Blaming, and Capability

Another way in which the social determinants of health are ignored takes the form of victim blaming. Many commentators, even those who see themselves as advocates of health, prefer to focus on what they call "personal responsibility" and dismiss the social context of people's lives. Certainly individual behaviors (such as, for example, smoking and alcohol) are an important determinant of health, as illustrated by the "Determinants of Health" model from *Healthy People 2010*. (Figure 3.2)[10] However, this model also illustrates all the other factors impacting upon health. The implication is that since many people (usually including those making these comments) eat right, exercise, don't smoke, and so on, that those who do are guilty and should have to suffer the consequences of this lack of responsibility.

Figure 3.2

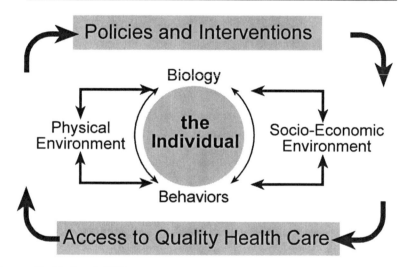

Determinants of Health

Source: *Healthy People* 2010

A typical presentation of the arguments for "personality responsibility" was made by John Mackey, the CEO of Whole Foods, Inc., in a *Wall Street Journal* op-ed arguing against the Affordable Care Act (ACA) and presenting the "Whole Foods alternative to Obamacare." Mackey presents "eight things that we can do", but are primarily suggestions for changes to insurance. The main feature of his proposals is inequity, because it rewards those who already have the resources to adopt and maintain behaviors that make them healthier. His proposals would increase the wealth of those who already have the most of it. This proposal, if implemented, would create enormous increases in insurance company profit, would not meet the health needs of those who have needs, and would end up costing a fortune. He talks about a balance between "controls" and "freedom" but the "controls" he describes are all on services that would benefit people, while the "freedom" is all for corporations to continue to have unfettered access to excessive profit. He argues that:

Unfortunately many of our health-care problems are self-inflicted: two-thirds of Americans are now overweight and one-third are obese. Most of the diseases that kill us and account for about 70% of all health-care spending—heart disease, cancer, stroke, diabetes and obesity—are mostly preventable through proper diet, exercise, not smoking, minimal alcohol consumption and other healthy lifestyle choices.[11]

Eat nutritious food, exercise, don't smoke or take illegal drugs or drink to excess, etc. This is good advice, and all of us should try to take it. I'm sure that it is advice that many of the employees of Whole Foods—the ones who are young and healthy—appreciate, because it validates what they do, and see—the "outcome" is that they are young and healthy. It is possible that there are other Whole Foods employees, not young and healthy but older and/or with chronic disease—who may not find his advice, or the company's health plan, to be of such great value. His essay may be a call to action for those who, given some combination of youth, genetic luck, good health, and socioeconomic opportunity, are still not doing all they can. But, as the Determinants of Health model makes clear, the ability of people to adopt healthful behaviors as individuals is very much affected by their environment. Where do they live? Is there a food store (forget a Whole Foods!) that they can walk to if they do not have a car? Is it safe from both predators and cars—are there sidewalks? Is there a factory spewing pollution or a toxic landfill or brownfield nearby? Where can their children play?

Whole Foods itself is built on the idea of providing nutritious food—to those who can afford it. Many Americans cannot; to try to purchase food there on food stamps would be insanity. What people who are young, healthy, rich, or a combination of all of these can do (and should do) is not necessarily an easy, or even viable, option for those without such privileges.

Mackey's op-ed attacks the "socialism" of the plan for Obamacare, and indeed begins with an epigram from Margaret Thatcher, "The problem with socialism is that eventually you run out of other people's money." Our health system, however, is expensive because of both the overuse of expensive technologies and the huge profits made by providers, drug companies, and insurers. Indeed, the most cost-effective part of our health system is Medicare, the health care insurance program for the elderly, which is the object of Mackey's attacks.

While I haven't done an analysis of the income levels of Whole Food shoppers, it's easy to see by the high prices, top quality food and a casual glance at their clientele that they don't cater to the poor. Their clients likely have better social determinants of health than lower-class Americans, which raises an interesting question: do these shoppers eat well because they have better social determinants, or do they have better social determinants (are wealthier) because they have made a personal decision to eat better? I have no idea what Mackey might answer to this question, but it's pretty obvious that the stores are not full of Horatio Alger types, now wealthy because they decided to eat organic. My point is that social determinants largely impact health choices, including limiting them to crappy cheap food that isn't good for your health. Yes, people need to eat better. And yes, they have some control over those choices. But the biggest factor to help them get there may be to make them wealthier, not excoriate them for eating junk food.

This is illustrated by the story of the bodies floating down the river that is told in Chapter 1. Problems are best addressed, when possible, by prevention. In Dr. Jones' "cliff analogy", the face of the cliff represents our medical care system. Activities carried out there are very costly; they may be very efficient at doing what they can do, but are very ineffective in terms of increasing health. When someone finally says "maybe we should go look upstream, and find out what's killing these people and causing them to fall into the river, and see if we can do something about it", they are suggesting that we move to the top of Dr. Jones' cliff; they are suggesting moving people back from the edge of the cliff. It is what is called, based on this analogy, "working upstream." Mr. Mackey's call for people to live healthier lives and adopt healthier behaviors is a call for upstream change, and is fine as far as it goes, but it is overly simplistic and looks at only one aspect of prevention, that of personal choice. It is great for those who can implement the behaviors he suggest, but at best it is limited because it doesn't address the issues that make it difficult for people to adopt such behaviors and at worst it is self-serving, self-justifying, and victim blaming. By focusing our concerns on personal choice, we obscure more effective discussions about how we change the social determinants that control the context in which better choices could be made. Telling unemployed people on food stamps and others struggling to make ends meet that they should spend more on food just doesn't count as effective policy making.

Why is it difficult for some individuals to adopt healthful behaviors? The concept of "capability", originally developed by Nobel Prize-winning economist Amartya Sen, and developed for use in health by Jennifer Prah Ruger[12], goes beyond simply evaluating people's behaviors. It looks at people's opportunity to perform those behaviors, which is not equally available to all. Whether one thinks that finding an hour a day to walk should be within the capability of anyone, the reality is that the vast majority of people do not begin to approach 60 minutes a day of exercise. For someone working two jobs, or living in a neighborhood that is dangerous or has no sidewalks, or who has no car to get to a park, that challenge is greater. In a plenary address to the Society of Teachers of Family Medicine, Robert Ferrer put it pithily: "The choices that people make are dependent upon the choices that they have."[13]

Capability is influenced by individual, social, psychological and environmental factors, as well as by income. While money—or lack of it—is a major factor, it is not the only one; other circumstances can mitigate or exacerbate financial issues. The concept of "social capital" developed by Robert Putnam in *Bowling Alone*[14], as well as by others, is one formulation of this. In his book *Heat Wave*, Eric Klinenberg describes how the deaths in the 1995 Chicago heat wave, while associated with age, illness, poverty and the availability of air-conditioning, were also associated with the availability of social supports. He notes the differential death rates in two adjacent low-income communities. In one, the decimation of the commercial sector and fear of crime had at-risk people locked in hot apartments, while in the other neighbors checked on the old, sick, and poor, and merchants on the vibrant shopping street allowed them access to their air-conditioned stores.[15]

In a 2010 article in *Annals of Family Medicine*, Drs. Ferrer and Alejandra Carrasco comment:

A capability perspective implies that poverty should not be defined primarily by income but by scarce opportunity to pursue valued activities and goals. Strong external supports create opportunities that enable people with limited income to pursue their goals for healthy living. Capability is thus a key mediator of the relationship between socioeconomic position and outcomes.[16]

What Ferrer and Carrasco add to the capability model introduced by Sen and developed by Prah Ruger is the clinical component. They show how the clinical relationship can take capability into account, and how the clinician can play a role in enhancing the health of patients through understanding and acting to help ameliorate the impact on those with low capability. They suggest, as an example, a series of questions that a clinician can ask in order to assess an individual's capability of adopting different healthful behaviors. They also provide suggestions for how the clinician or practice can access help through social service agencies, public health departments, programs of connectors or promotores, and grass-roots agencies. Clinicians may be able to assist in helping people gain access to wholesome food or places to exercise, and to groups that would support their activities.

Addressing Health Inequities and the
Social Determinants of Health

While the term "health disparities" is the "official" one used by the U.S. government, a more accurate term (commonly used in Europe) is health inequities. Disparities means differences, but inequities means that one of the "different" groups is worse off. It also makes clear that these differences in health status are not "just there" or that they result from the inexorable ravages of time like the health difference between young and old, but rather result from "treatable" differences in social situations; this ties them clearly to issues of social justice. These are things that we can do something about, even if it is not easy.

In 2011, Michael Marmot served as President of the British Medical Association (BMA). During his tenure the BMA published *Social Determinants of Health: What Doctors Can Do*[17], which presents conceptual models and large-scale goals, as well as principled statements of how physicians must act to create conditions of social justice and reduce the gradient of health disparity that results from different life circumstance. For example, it takes from Marmot's book *Fair Society, Healthy Lives* the following set of policy objectives that physicians and their organizations should work towards: [18]

A. Give every child the best start in life
B. Enable all children, young people and adults to maximize their capabilities and have control over their lives
C. Create fair employment and good work for all
D. Ensure healthy standard of living for all

E. Create and develop healthy and sustainable places and communities

F. Strengthen the role and impact of ill health prevention

One example that the report develops in greater depth is for "cold housing." It cites the existing data on the direct impact of cold housing on health:

- Countries which have more energy efficient housing have lower excess winter deaths (EWDs).
- EWDs are almost three times higher in the coldest quarter of housing than in the warmest quarter.
- Around 40% of EWDs are attributable to cardiovascular diseases.
- Around 33% of EWDs are attributable to respiratory diseases.
- Mental health is negatively affected by fuel poverty and cold housing for any age group.
- Cold housing increases the level of minor illnesses such as colds and flu and exacerbates existing conditions such as arthritis and rheumatism.
- Cold housing negatively affects dexterity and increases the risk of accidents and injuries in the home.

It also notes the indirect impacts:

- Cold housing negatively affects children's educational attainment, emotional well-being and resilience.
- Fuel poverty negatively affects dietary opportunities and choices.
- Investing in the energy efficiency of housing can help stimulate the labour market and economy, as well as creating opportunities for skilling up the construction workforce.

This provides a thorough, evidence-based, and very sobering portrayal by a major medical association of the health consequences of what is not normally considered a "medical" problem. Beyond identifying the problem, the BMA identified places and programs that were effectively addressing them. They created—and are continuing to add to—a searchable database, so other communities can benefit from the findings.

What are some of the components of the social determinants of health? They include, certainly, housing, food, warmth, education, the overall treatment of women and especially the education of women. The unequal distribution of these components of the social determinants of health is a major cause of health disparities, which is the term used by *Healthy People 2020* for the variances in health status among populations of people that are amenable to change, that exists because people live at different places along the cliff, and would be decreased or eliminated if the people who are most at risk could be moved further from the cliff face.

One way to illustrate how social circumstances influence health is to look at the causes of death in the U.S., not by the traditional method of listing the end-stage disease (cardiovascular disease, cancer, stroke, pneumonia, liver disease) but rather the underlying causes, as presented in Table 3.1. Developed by Steven Woolf and his group at the Virginia Commonwealth University, it presents a list of the 9 most common etiologies of death, from tobacco use (400,000 deaths per year) through illicit drugs (20,000). Seen this way, by root cause, we get a clearer picture of the true role of social determinants. Only one item on the list (#4, microbial agents), is even considered part of traditional medicine.

Educational level, along with socioeconomic status, is probably the best predictor of health status. The Commission on

Table 3.1

Real Causes of Death in the U.S.

Etiologic Agent	# deaths per year
Tobacco use	400,000
Diet/activity	300,000
Alcohol	100,000
Microbial agents	90,000
Toxic Agents	60,000
Firearms	35,000
Sexual behaviors	30,000
Motor vehicles	25,000
Illicit use of drugs*	20,000

Source: Personal communication, Steven Woolf, M.D.

Health of the Robert Wood Johnson Foundation provides a stunning series of graphs showing that more education is associated with longer lives for both men and women and each racial/ethnic group. Higher parental level of education is tied to lower infant mortality and better health of their children. They propose three pathways through which education impacts on health: through health knowledge and behaviors, through workplace risks, and through social standing and stress[19].

Woolf and his colleagues present a provocative "thought experiment,"[20] demonstrating that even if we attribute all current and recent reduction in mortality to medical advances (nowhere near true; most are due to the types of societal change generally characterized as "public health", such as clean water, sanitation, and cleaner air), the impact of eliminating the disparities that exist on the basis of educational level would have an effect that was several times as large as the impact of medical advances. More lives would be saved by education than all of medical advances.

The differences in even slight variations in these social determinants can be rigorously calculated—with an actual interactive calculator, sometimes providing shocking results. The County Health Calculator produced by Woolf and colleagues is available free online.[21] For those interested in public health issues, it is the medical equivalent of a service such as Zillow, but instead of looking up your estimated home value, you can see health stats for your county (and any county). It allows one to look at the socioeconomic status (measured as a percent of people with incomes >200% of poverty) and education (measured as a percent of people with at least some college) for every state and county, and compare it to the other states, or to counties within a state. A neat "slider" feature allows you to change these rates (e.g., make the rate the same as the best or worst) and see what the change in deaths would be. For example, in Harris County, Texas (Houston), if 5% more people attended some college and 5% more had an income higher than twice the federal poverty level we could expect to save 1,200 lives, prevent 12,200 cases of diabetes, and eliminate $97.8 million in diabetes costs every year.

Elizabeth Bradley and colleagues challenge the simplicity of the notion that the U.S. spends far more per capita on health care than other developed countries. While certainly true, the U.S. also spends far less on social services that might decrease the need for health care; when lumped together, the difference decreases. The OECD average was about 1.7 times as much spending on social services as health care, with New Zealand leading at about 2.6. The U.S. stands out as being one of only 3 countries (along with Mexico and Korea) which spends less on social services than health care and where most of the combined health and social services spending is on medical care.[22] In other words, ensuring that the most disadvantaged have their basic needs (housing, food, education, safety, etc.), addressing the social determinants of health, having policies that create a more equitable and just society, has a major impact on health status.

As I have indicated earlier, health status in the U.S. is impacted by two major factors. One, because our healthcare system is built on private insurance, profit, and high-technology rather than primary care (all of which will be discussed in future chapters), many people do not have access to health care, or receive inappropriate and even harmful care. The other is the social determinants of health, the social conditions that make people who are less well-off more likely to be sick or have other potential health problems (like unintended pregnancy).

Is this a big or a small problem? How does it impact the overall status of health in the U.S.? Is it getting better or worse? "The State of U.S. Health, 1990-2010: Burden of Diseases, Injuries, and Risk Factors,"[23] written by the members of the U.S. Burden of Disease Collaboration, an enormous group of population-health scholars from institutions across the country and a few from other parts of the world, describes the state of health in the U.S. over that 20-year period, and compares it to the other 33 "developed" countries in the Organization for Economic Cooperation and Development (OECD).

The main results show that, since 1990, the health status of the U.S. has improved in most areas:

- Average life expectancy has increased,
  from 75.2 to 78.2 years;
- Healthy life expectancy (HALE) has increased,
  from 65.8 to 68.1 years.

These are good things; that is, they are moving in the right direction, although more recent evidence shows that for at least one group, women, and especially non-Hispanic white women, mortality rates are actually getting worse.[24] However, even for other groups, they are moving in the right direction more slowly than in the other OECD countries. Since 1990, the U.S. rank for life expectancy (at birth) has dropped from 20th to 27th among these 34 countries, and the HALE has dropped from 14th to 26th. If other countries are rapidly outpacing us, we are surely not doing all we could.

There are a few more terms used in the report, probably unfamiliar but not that hard to understand: Life expectancy is decreased by the years of life lost (YLL) through premature (age-standardized) death due to disease or injury. The difference between absolute life expectancy and HALE is the number of years lived with disability (YLD). The sum of YLL and YLD is expressed as disability-adjusted life years (DALY), kind of the complement of HALE. That is, the lower the DALY, the fewer years of life have been either lost to premature death or lived with disability.

From 1990, the U.S. rank among the OECD countries has dropped in all these areas:

- From 18th to 27th in age-standardized death rate;
- From 23rd to 28th in YLL;
- From 5th to 6th in age-standardized YLD.

These are not good things. The publication includes a table that provides, for each of the 34 countries studied, the rank for YLL for each of 25 conditions: green means significantly better than the mean, yellow about the mean, and red significantly worse. The U.S. is green in only one (stroke), and is red in 15.

The other important thing done by the study's authors was to look at risk factors for YLL and YLD in the U.S. It is easier to measure mortality (death) than morbidity (disability), but the latter is very important because, as noted in the abstract, "As the U.S. population has aged, YLDs have comprised a larger share of DALYs than YLLs." That is, years lived with disability exceeds years of life lost from treatable disease. This makes sense; as we have developed increasingly sophisticated (and costly) high-tech interventions to prevent death, we have increased the number of years that people are kept alive but suffering from the symptoms and complications of their diseases.

The diseases and injuries with the largest number of YLLs in 2010 were ischemic heart disease, lung cancer, stroke, chronic obstructive pulmonary disease, and road injury. Age-standardized YLL rates increased for Alzheimer disease, drug use disorders, chronic kidney disease, kidney cancer, and falls. The diseases with the largest number of YLDs in 2010 were low back pain, major depressive disorder, other musculoskeletal disorders, neck pain, and anxiety disorders. The leading risk factors related to DALYs were dietary risks, tobacco smoking, high body mass index, high blood pressure, high fasting plasma glucose, physical inactivity, and alcohol use.

The largest number of YLLs were caused by the "traditional" chronic diseases, and most of the conditions that caused an increase in YLL over the last 20 years were those that one would expect to increase as we keep people alive longer, particularly Alzheimer's disease, chronic kidney disease, falls, and drug use disorders. This last includes not just "illicit" or "illegal" drug use, but use of prescription drugs, in particular for chronic pain. Not coincidentally, the conditions for which these drugs are used comprise a large proportion of the diseases that have the largest number of YLDs—back pain, other musculoskeletal disorders, and neck pain.

These findings should guide our population/public health interventions. The leading risk factors for DALYs are not surprising; they are the ones that we hear about all the time. These are the very areas, in fact, where most population/public health programs are currently focused. However, when it comes to public policy, laws, and spending money to try to solve the problems, we are woefully deficient in the U.S. There has been some success in the regulation of smoking in public places, although not without significant resistance from those who profit from tobacco, including the tobacco industry, tobacco retailers, and clubs and casinos. Public health interventions in the other areas have had much greater opposition (such as New York City's efforts to limit portion size of sugar-filled soft drinks), or the interventions are non-existent.

If, as demonstrated by Steven Woolf and others, the gaps—inequities—in health status were to be closed, if everyone had the same health status as upper middle class whites (as noted previously, the longevity for poor white women is dropping), if everyone had the same health status as those with even some college, if everyone had the same health status as those with an income as little as twice the federal poverty level, the number of lives saved would be enormous. It would far exceed all the health benefits of traditional "public health" programs (clean water supply and seatbelts in motor vehicles, for two major examples), which themselves account for much more health benefit than medical care.

What is popular, rather than implementing programs aimed at improving the social determinants of health, is victim-blaming: telling people who are overweight, inactive, smokers, drinkers, and victims of diabetes or hypertension to "clean up their acts", to stop, to lose weight, to adopt healthy habits. Of course, these are good things to do, and we see increasing numbers of individuals doing them. However, the success rate is much higher among groups with higher income and higher educational levels, which must mean something. It could be that they know that smoking, obesity, inactivity, drinking, drugs, and not taking medicine for diabetes and high blood pressure are bad for you, while poorer people don't. That, however, is hard to imagine. It is more likely due to their greater resources to try to address these problems, social support for healthful behaviors (including jobs), and access to health care. In addition, the same interests that lobby against regulation of smoking, unhealthy foods and alcohol are heavily advertising these same substances in the least-advantaged communities.

These are "social determinants of health." It is not only access to health care, but safe communities, stable housing, education, and prospects for jobs—the very things that national and often state policymakers seem to be least willing to fund, and the areas that other OECD countries often do fund. Bradley and Taylor, in their New York Times op-ed "To fix health care, help the poor,"[25] discuss their scientific paper that demonstrates that the U.S. stands out among OECD countries in that the vast majority of its combined health and social services spending is on medical care. This helps explain both our decrease in YLL caused by treatable but essentially end-stage medical conditions and our increase in YLD and in risk factors for chronic disease, because we do not treat the "upstream" circumstances of people's lives that lead to "downstream" disability and death.

It is not about the money. As a nation, we have the money. It is, as I have said before, about the will. It is about the will of politicians, who are ideologically committed to the principle that the only ones who really deserve government assistance are the largest corporations and wealthiest individuals. Politicians who have, as *New York Times* columnist Charles Blow has said, a gag reflex to the word "social."[26] If we are to have a healthy society, we need to address the social determinants of health. Doctors and other professionals must consider social conditions that cause poor health to be part of their mandate and work to change them. All of us must hold our leaders responsible for policies that promote health, or make it worse, including ensuring that all of us have our basic human needs met.

A significant strategy to address social determinants and health disparities is the implementation of "health in all" policies, for such things as:

- Land use (what is the density? Are there open spaces? How is space used?)
- Built environment (are distances to schools and shopping walkable? Are there facilities for exercise?)
- Transportation (can people get to the store or the park?)
- Agriculture (what about antibiotic and drug use in raising livestock? How about the conditions of farmworkers, includ-

ing exposure to pesticides?)

- Environmental Justice (are there toxins in the environment? Lead? Who is exposed to "brownfields" and do their children have higher rates of cancer?)
- Health policies (smoking in public places)
- Taxes (do these encourage or discourage the building of a healthful society?)

A society can never achieve a significant improvement in health, or decrease health disparities, unless it consciously and forthrightly addresses the social determinants of health. Although these areas are outside of traditional medicine, physicians and other health professionals can be involved in addressing them; they are community leaders who have great potential moral authority, and it is better to be involved in these efforts rather than sit comfortably in our offices and hospitals tending to the individual health problems of people that could have been prevented.

The important point is that health care providers, including physicians, should not be casting blame on the victims of ill health but can and should be involved in advocating for the societal changes that will enhance people's health and increase their capability. In 1848, Virchow wrote in his report that:

Physicians are the natural advocates of the poor, and social problems fall to a large extent within their jurisdiction . . . medicine has imperceptibly led us into the social field and placed us in a position of confronting directly the great problems of our time.[27]

This is still true in our time.

References

1. Hart, JT. The inverse care law. *The Lancet.* 297:7696, 405-412, 1971.
2. Virchow, RC. Report on the Typhus Epidemic in Upper Silesia. *Am J Public Health,* 96(12): 2102-2105, 2006.
3. El Norte. https://en.wikipedia.org/wike/El Norte (film)
4. Ibid # 1.
5. The several hundred papers from the Whitehall studies can be found at: http://www.ucl.ad.uk/whitehallll/publications
6. Jones, CP, Jones, CY, Perry, GS. Addressing the social determinants of children's health: A cliff analogy. *J Health Care for the Poor and Underserved,* 20 (4): 1-12, 2009.
7. Centers for Disease Control, Health Disparities and Inequalities Report, United States, 2013.
8. Pear, R. Health law's pay policy is skewed, panel finds. *New York Times,* April 27, 2014.
9. Ibid # 8, Quoting Goodrich, K.
10. U.S. Department of Health and Human Services. *Healthy People 2010: Understanding and Improving Health,* 2nd ed. Washington, D.C.: U.S. Government Printing Office, November 2000.
11. Mackey, J. The Whole Foods alternative to Obamacare. *Wall Street Journal,* August 11, 2010.
12. Ruger, JP. Health capability: conceptualization and operationalization. *Am J Public Health* 100 (1): 41-49, January 2010.
13. Ferrer, R. Building a healthy commons. Plenary address to the Society of Teachers of Family Medicine Annual Conference, San Antonio, TX, May 2014.
14. Putnam, RD. *Bowling Alone: The Collapse and Revival of American Community,* New York. Simon & Schuster, 2000.
15. Klinenberg, E. *Heat Wave: A Social Autopsy of a Disaster in Chicago.* Chicago. University of Chicago Press, 2003.
16. Ferrer, RL, Carrasco, AV. Capability and clinical success. *Ann Fam Med* 8: 454-460, 2010.
17. Social determinants of health: What doctors can do. British Medical Association, October 2011. Accessible at htpp://bma.org.uk/search?query=social%20determinants%20of%20health
18. Marmot, M, Allen, J, Goldblatt, P et al. Fair Society, Healthy Lives: Strategic Re-

view of Health Inequalities in England post 2010. London.

19. Commission to build a healthier America. Issue Brief 6. Education and Health, Robert Wood Johnson Foundation, September 2009.

20. Woolf, SH, Johnson, RE, Phillips, RL Jr. et al. Giving everyone the health of the educated: an examination of whether social change would save more lives than medical advances. *Am J Public Health* 97 (4): 679-683, April 2007.

21. Woolf, SH, Jones, RM, Johnson, RE et al. Avertable deaths associated with household income in Virginia. *Am J Public Health* 100: 750-755, 2010. htpp://countyhealthcalculator.org/

22. Bradley, E, Elkins, BR, Herrin, J et al. Health and social services expenditures: associations with health outcomes. *Brit Med J Quality and Safety* 20(10): 826-831, October 2011.

23. U.S. Burden of Disease Collaborators. The State of U.S. Health 1990-2010. *JAMA.* Published on line July 10, 2013.

24. Kindig, DA, Cheng, ER. Even as mortality fell in most U.S. counties, female mortality nonetheless rose in 42.8 percent of counties from 1992 to 2006. *Health Affairs (Millwood)* 32(3): 451-458, 2013.

25. Bradley, EH, Taylor, L. To fix health, help the poor. *New York Times*, December 8, 2011.

26. Blow, C. Resonance resistant. *New York Times*, May 18, 2013.

27. Ibid # 2

Chapter 4:

Dead Man Walking: The Impact of the U.S. Health System on the Health of the Public

Mr. Davis had had an inkling that something was awry, but he'd been unable to pay for an evaluation. "If we'd found it sooner it would have made a difference. But now I'm just a dead man walking."[1]

—Stillman and Tailor

In the last chapter, I discussed the fact that different populations have different health status for reasons that go beyond access to health care. These differences are called health disparities, but because they are potentially remediable they are more properly termed inequities. For example, there are health differences, disparities, between the old and the young, but we cannot make people younger; however, disparities based on income, ethnicity and race, gender and sexual preference, and even geographic location are manifestations of inequity. These do not cause small problems at the edges of our society; they are a large part of the reason that our health status is so much worse than that of other developed countries, as detailed in Chapter 2. However, the impact of health inequities and our lack of attention to social determinants of health are only part of the story. In this chapter, I shall provide more detail on how much worse our health is, as a population, as a result of our health system. Our social and health structure is not benign; it creates and fosters such inequities and it takes a major toll on the health of our people.

At the 2013 Annual Meeting of the Association of American Medical Colleges (AAMC), the organization's director of health workforce studies reported its findings from a survey that asked people whether they had always, sometimes, or never seen a doctor when they felt they needed to within the last year. On a positive note, 85% said "always." Of course, that means 15%—a lot of people!—said "sometimes" (12%) or "never" (3%). Of those 15%, over half (56%) indicated the obstacle was financial, not having the money (or insurance). This is a problem, and it is one that the Affordable Care Act (ACA) was designed to remedy; it will help but will not completely address it. For starters, people who are undocumented will not be eligible for any coverage under the act, and there are at least 17 million of these folks.[2] Secondly, the decision of the Supreme Court to allow states to opt out of Medicaid expansion means that in those states people who were not previously Medicaid eligible and make less than 133% of the federal poverty level will remain uninsured. They are ineligible for subsidized insurance because the plan under ACA was to cover this portion of the population via Medicaid expansion.

This has created bizarre and heart-rending situations, most obvious in towns that straddle a state border, like Texarkana, whose residents on the Arkansas side are eligible for Medicaid while those on the Texas side are not.[3] Finally, there are many people who find that their costs are increasing because businesses are not covering them and the cost of insurance makes it unaffordable. The subsidies that exist for many under the ACA are passed on to private insurance companies, and often leave working people with costs that they cannot afford.

Of course, as former President George W. Bush famously said in July, 2007, "I mean, people have access to health care in America. After all, you just go to an emergency room."[4] There is general consensus that this is not a very good source of repeated care in terms of quality. Also, if you have had to use the ER regularly for your care and already have a huge unpaid stack of bills from them, it can make you reluctant to return. This likely contributes to the "sometimes" responses found in the AAMC study, which probably often mean "sometimes I can ride it out but sometimes I am so sick that I have to go even though I dread the financial result." Following this ER theme, Mitt Romney declared repeatedly during the 2012 Presidential campaign, that no one dies for lack of health insurance,[5] despite many studies to the contrary. And this despite the fact that as Governor of Massachusetts he presumably thought it was a big enough issue that he championed the passage in his state of what became the model for the federal Affordable Care Act.

People do, in fact, die for lack of health insurance. We'll review some real cases to see how lack of insurance can kill, and to understand some of the interplay of the social determinants of health that are the backdrop to emergency room visits. People may be able to go to the ER when they have symptoms, but the ER is for acute problems. Sometimes a person's illness is so far advanced by the time that they have symptoms severe enough to drive them to the ER that they *will* die, even though the problem might have been successfully treated if they had presented earlier. Or, the ER makes a diagnosis of a life-threatening problem, but the person's lack of insurance means that they will not be able to find follow-up care, particularly if that care is going to cost a lot of money (for example, the diagnosis and treatment of cancer).

Michael Stillman and Monalisa Tailor present a typical story in the *New England Journal of Medicine,* titled "Dead Man Walking"[6] (grab a tissue first):

> *We met Tommy Davis in our hospital's clinic for indigent persons in March 2013 (the name and date have been changed to protect the patient's privacy). He and his wife had been chronically uninsured despite working full-time jobs and were now facing disastrous consequences.*
>
> *The week before this appointment, Mr. Davis had come to our emergency department with abdominal pain and obstipation. His examination, laboratory tests, and CT scan had cost him $10,000 (his entire life savings), and at evening's end he'd been sent home with a diagnosis of metastatic colon cancer.*
>
> *Mr. Davis had had an inkling that something was awry, but he'd been unable to pay for an evaluation... "If we'd found it sooner," he contended, "it would have made a difference. But now I'm just a dead man walking."[6]*

The story, in fact, gets worse. And it is only one story. There are many, many others, just in the experience of these two physicians. "Seventy percent of our clinic patients have no health insurance, and they are all frighteningly vulnerable; their care is erratic." And the authors are just two doctors, in a state that is taking advantage of the Supreme Court decision on the ACA to avoid expanding Medicaid.

This same theme is reflected in a front-page piece in the *New York Times*:

> *Late last month, Donna Atkins, a waitress at a barbecue restaurant, learned from Dr. Guy Petruzzelli, a surgeon here, that she has throat cancer. She does not have insurance and had a sore throat for a year before going to a doctor. She was advised to get a specialized image of her neck, but it would have cost $2,300, more than she makes in a month. "I didn't have the money even to walk in the door of that office," said Ms. Atkins.* [7]

These problems are everywhere, as was brought home to me very starkly when I recently served as the attending physician on our inpatient service in the hospital. We take care of a lot of patients, and they are very sick. Their medical diagnoses varied: kidney failure, diabetic ketoacidosis, malignant hypertension, severe asthma exacerbation, infections in a variety of places, etc. But, really, the most common diagnosis was lack of access to health care, mainly because of lack of health insurance. While not all these people are poor, they, like most people, have limited incomes, and have many other basic needs (rent, food, caring for their children) that compete with health care for the dollars available. Asymptomatic diseases (or conditions with "tolerable" symptoms) often seem to be a lower priority.

I'd like to share some of their stories, although obviously I cannot share their names or present too many actual details about them; I'll make up initials and change some details that do not affect the essential issues. These are real people, with real names and real problems.

AG has diabetes and high blood pressure. (These two conditions, diabetes and high blood pressure, are going to be a recurrent theme; they are the mainstay, most-common, diseases of any general adult medicine practice. They are treatable, but when not well controlled their complications—strokes or kidney failure or heart attacks or amputations—are also major contributors to the work of many subspecialists: cardiologists and endocrinologists and nephrologists and neurologists and surgeons and orthopedists, just to name a few.) AG had lost his job, and while unemployed and without health insurance he hadn't been going to the doctor. Luckily, his chronic diseases weren't bothering him much, except for a small sore on the bottom of his foot. High blood pressure often causes no symptoms, until the stroke or heart attack; foot sores in diabetes are a big threat, because the disease both diminishes the sensation of pain, so it doesn't hurt much, and the fact that diabetes causes poor circulation of blood means that it doesn't heal well, but the lack of pain makes it seem not so bad. He finally found a job, a reasonably good job with the promise of health insurance after a while. Unfortunately, it involved walking almost 20 miles per day, not a good thing for his foot. The foot developed a severe infection, requiring expensive hospitalization for intravenous antibiotics, and might still need to be amputated.

PS also has diabetes, which, especially when untreated, makes one susceptible to infections, and he has had several of them. Now, in late middle age, he presents with a very serious infection, requiring not only intravenous antibiotics, but surgery to clean out the pus, resulting in an open wound. A machine attached to drain out the residual infection and keep it clean will need to be regularly replaced for many weeks as he continues the intravenous antibiotics. Fortunately (should you ever be in a similar situation), home health can be arranged to provide these services. Provided, that is, you have health insurance coverage. Oh yes, and a home. PS has neither. This makes follow-up care a little more difficult.

DR is a good deal younger but also had a severe infection requiring long-term antibiotics for a foot infection, after an unsuccessful attempt at outpatient treatment. And, yes, his diabetes is uncontrolled because he hasn't had insurance and so hasn't gone to the doctor or taken his medicine in quite a while. He also had lost over 80% of his kidney function, so he'll be on dialysis soon. There is a "silver lining" (!); thanks to a law passed early in the 1970s, anyone with end-stage kidney disease requiring dialysis is eligible for Medicare, so he will be insured. Of course, the cost to Medicare will be far, far more than would have been the treatment of his diabetes, had he had coverage before the "end stage."

MT will also become insured through this wonderful program, although her kidney failure is due mainly to untreated high blood pressure rather than diabetes. As I noted above, high blood pressure is often asymptomatic (thus the sobriquet "silent killer"); she didn't have insurance or mon-

ey so didn't go to the doctor to find out how uncontrolled it was, as it slowly destroyed her kidneys.

Not all of our patients' problems came from diabetes or infections, and not everyone who is uninsured is poor.

KF has asthma, pretty severe asthma, for which he was taking an inhaler to be able to breathe. It is a bronchodilator (airway-opener), the right drug for an acute attack, but KF's attack never went away and he was taking far more of it than was safe. And spending an awful lot of money on it. It is available for a much lower cost at some pharmacies that provide certain generic medications for $4, but he didn't know that. He does now, after being in the hospital for a week getting expensive breathing treatments. It's a good thing, too, because the other inhalers that he needs to prevent (or at least decrease the frequency and severity of) these attacks, steroids and sustained-release bronchodilators, cost a lot, well over $100 per inhaler. They have been around for a long time, so one would expect that by now at least some of them would be available generically and cheaper. But there's a fascinating story here. The propellant in these inhalers used to be fluorocarbons, but these, as we know, destroy the ozone layer and contribute to a lot of bad environmental effects. So they were made illegal, and the pharmaceutical manufacturers had to replace them with environmentally safe propellants. Good for the environment. Unfortunately, it's bad for KF and millions of other people with asthma; using a different propellant meant that the drug was a "new formulation", which allowed the drug makers to extend their patents for many years. So, low-cost *inhaled steroids are still not available. This sounds like a cruel joke, but it is not a joke. The pharmaceutical companies will not suffer; only patients will.*

These five people were cared for in one week, on one hospital service, in one hospital, and they were not the only ones with a primary diagnosis of lack of health insurance coverage. Of course, we also took care of lots of sick people with health insurance. People with insurance, even with good insurance, also get serious diseases and need to be hospitalized. But these people stand out because they didn't have to be as sick as they were or require the costly services that they did. Their predicament is the result of their social standing and socioeconomic position, the result of health inequities. That they were in this situation is not only immoral and bad medicine, it is bad economics. It is inexcusable.

There is a good chance that some of these people will be able to buy affordable, subsidized insurance through the federally-run exchange in my state. However, given that most of them likely make less than 133% of the poverty level, which means they were supposed to be covered by expanded Medicaid, they are out of luck because my state, Kansas, has refused Medicaid expansion. And, although Kansas City straddles a state line like Texarkana, they are further out of luck because Missouri has also not expanded Medicaid. And even if they get insurance, it will not touch the other negative determinants of health; it will not, for example, get PS a home.

A few years after Hurricane Katrina, I was in a still-devastated New Orleans, and came across a building with a sign on the side: Tulane Community Health Center at Covenant House. I was pleased that there was such a center, because there was—and remains—great need. But I was surprised to continue reading "Sustained through a generous gift from the People of Qatar." And under it: "Qatar Katrina Fund." I admit to being shocked.

Yes, it is very generous of the People of Qatar. I am certain that the Tulane Community Health Center is providing vital health care services to the people of that community thanks to the funds from the People of Qatar. But it is sad that in the "richest country in the world", the home of all those multibillionaire financiers and bankers who were still rich, even after the near-collapse of the economy in 2008, people must rely on the generosity of the people of Qatar to fund a clinic in one of its own cities, several years after a major natural disaster. Many in the U.S. rail against providing "foreign aid" (much of it munitions) to other countries, but our poor are recipients of international foreign aid for health care because we, as a nation, will not meet their basic health needs.

The desperate search that many people have for health care is illustrated by the regular enormous turnouts that occur at episodic regional "free clinics" such as those sponsored by the National Association of Free Clinics. Staffed with volunteer nurses, physicians, other health professionals and lay people who help with the organization, these clinics are massively attended. At one such event in Kansas City, over 1,000 people showed up on a day when the temperature was less than 20 degrees and the roads were still covered with ice from the snow the night before. People were treated, for acute conditions including pneumonia and for chronic diseases such as high blood pressure, diabetes, high cholesterol and others that they may have been aware of for years but were unable to afford treatment for, and unable to see a physician. Most of these people are not homeless, destitute or even unemployed. They work in low-wage jobs without health insurance, and often come from rural areas where even the existing free clinics in cities are inaccessible because of distance. "Making $3 an hour plus tips I can't afford to see a doctor," one person told the newspaper, "When you have your house payments and your bills, it is hard." And it is hard when you can only pay for 4 things and you and your family need, really *need,* 5 or 6 or 7. It is hard in a way that most of our more well-to-do may never know. Many working people are only a few paychecks away from this situation. A recent study asked a random sample of Americans "How confident are you that you could come up with $2,000 if an unexpected need arose within the next month?" The result: "Almost 40% of individuals in the United States either could not or probably could not come up with even $2,000 if an unexpected need arose."[8]

That people can get treatment at events such as those mass episodic clinics is nice, but it neither solves the health problem for the individual, who will need ongoing care, or of our society, which will continue to have a large percentage of its population chronically ill, undertreated, and often unable to work. These large events are very like the international trips (often called "mission trips" even when they are not focused on religious evangelism) that doctors and medical students make to many underdeveloped countries. Sometimes they do discrete procedures, such as when otolaryngologists (ear, nose and throat, ENT, surgeons) do a large number of cleft palate repairs in a short time. These can be great, and lifesavers, especially if the patients can get reasonable follow-up care. Sometimes these trips provide primary care, diagnosis and possibly some treatment of acute and chronic disease. Sometimes they find a serious problem, say an obvious cancer. In those instances, where complex long term care is needed, there is often no treatment.

Primary care and chronic disease care cannot be done successfully in a mass, one-time or very intermittent manner, whether internationally or in the U.S. It is unfortunate that there are such desperately needy people in the world. To address this problem, many international medical organizations such as Partners in Health, Doctors Without Borders, and Doctors for Global Health have recognized that the solution is infrastructure and continuity of care, not episodic visits. In the U.S., it is more than unfortunate. It is unacceptable; we have the resources, and yet our leaders are thus far unwilling to deploy them.

Access to health care need not be tied to socioeconomic status, and in most wealthy countries it isn't. (Examples include Canada, the United Kingdom, France, Switzerland, etc.) The social determinants of health still exist in those countries, and poor people have to struggle (although the global social support structure in most such countries is far more developed than in the U.S.) but paying for health care is not an issue. The French movie *Le Havre* features an older male protagonist who shines shoes at the port; he and his wife are poor. They live in a tiny house off an alley, have no phone and no car. One day his wife is stricken with severe illness, and is hospitalized for weeks. It is a fictional story, but my point is not a focus of the story, but what is not even mentioned. These people, director Aki Kaurismäki makes clear, have very little and are never certain if he will earn enough to buy food for dinner. When she needs to go to the hospital, he goes to the closest phone, in a store some distance away, and is lucky enough to obtain a ride for her to the hospital from the woman at the store. But there is not a line, not a word, in the film, about how they will pay for a hospitalization that lasts weeks. It is not part of the story because it is simply not an issue in France; health care is covered. In the U.S., any man coming home to find his wife collapsed would of course get her to the hospital without thinking right then about the cost. But all too soon it would become a big concern; it is impossible in the U.S. not to ponder how one would pay for health care in such a crisis. The fact that this is so is a scandal. Our system is not designed to provide people with access to care, either financially or in terms of providing a primary care medical infrastructure that can see them.

In Chapter 5, on Primary Care, I present a graphic from the Robert Graham Center that shows the increased number of physicians that the U.S. will need going forward. This is mostly a result of population growth but also from the aging of that population, along with a one-time jump because of the increased numbers of people who will be insured as a result of the ACA (although this will have to be adjusted down in the future because of the states that are not expanding Medicaid). Just from population growth and aging, we will require about 64,000 more physicians by 2025. In addition, the one-time jump because of the ACA is about 27,000, bringing the total number of additional physicians that we will require to 91,000.

There is a big problem here. That we will need more doctors because we have more people, or because our population is aging and older people require more medical care, is one thing. But the need for more doctors because more people will be insured is disturbing. Those people are already here now; they get sick, and they need care *now,* no less than they will when and if they are covered in the future. It is ironic that we now realize we have a shortage of doctors because more people will have insurance; they needed to have doctors anyway. That this situation existed is an example of inequity and injustice.

The Myths and Realities of Emergency Room "Over Use"

Often, people in the situation of Tommy Davis, described above, have gone to the emergency room for their care, as President George W. Bush suggested. Sometimes, as in his case, it is too late. It is common for health policy analysts to bemoan the "overuse" of emergency departments for primary care, largely because the cost is so much higher and care could be delivered so much more appropriately in an office visit. So why did Mr. Davis, and why do so many others, use the emergency room for primary care? Clearly, a big part of it is financial, as noted by the AAMC study. But some of it is perceptual. People who are poor, uninsured, underinsured, and unempowered often prefer the emergency room to seeking primary care in doctors' offices. One possible explanation could be that they feel accepted in that setting, like it is "their" place, unlike the physician's office. There also are concrete and logical reasons.

In an effort to identify those reasons, Shreya Kangovi and colleagues analyzed interviews with frequent emergency room users in Philadelphia about their reasons for doing so. Most of the subjects were lower income African Americans. The interviews were conducted using trained community members to engender greater trust on the part of the patients.[9]

Study respondents (both the insured and uninsured) explained that they consciously chose the ER because the care was cheaper, the quality of care was seemingly better, transportation options were more readily accessible, and, in some cases, the hospital offered more respite than a physician's office.

These findings should be surprising to many students of public policy, but they were the legitimate perspectives of the people who were using these services, those Kangovi correctly notes, whose *"...voices are seldom heard in policy discussions."* Understanding their concerns is critical, not because they are always "right", or represent everyone, but because those concerns reflect their experiences, and the degree to which our current strategies are not working, and the degree to which our future strategies are unlikely to work if they do not take into consideration what motivates people to use emergency rooms. Three themes generated by the researchers stood out, accompanied by supporting quotes from the folks who were interviewed:

Convenience: "You must call on the same day to set up a [primary] care appointment ... whenever they can fit you in." This open-access scheduling resulted in people taking days off from work and still being unable to see a doctor. It also made it impossible for many to access transportation covered by Medicaid because the transport arrangements had to made 72 hours in advance. Late hospital hours also made care more available.

Cost: "I don't have a co-pay in the ER, but my primary [physician] may send me to two or three specialists and sometimes there is a co-pay for them. Plus there's time off from work to go to several appointments."

Quality: "The [primary care doctor] never treated me or my husband aggressively to get blood pressure under control. I went to the hospital and they had it under control in four days. The [physician] had three years."

Any health care provider who has worked in an ER or in ambulatory care can validate these concerns, and also respond to them. Cost is the most clear-cut. Obviously care in an ER is not free; indeed, as noted above, the cost of emergency care is a major driver of efforts to get people to *not* use it. But the patient, at the time of service, doesn't have to put down cash, put down a co-payment, or put down real money now. There will be a bill, but that will come later and be something that goes on their (likely existing and mounting) debt burden. Or, if they have Medicaid, it may be paid for by the government. In the meantime, the ER, unlike most physicians' offices, will see them (indeed, has to under a federal law called the Emergency Medical Treatment and Labor Act, EMTALA).

Convenience is, perhaps, a poor choice of words; it suggests something purely volitional, as if people were choosing to have their hair done during the day rather than go to the doctor. Convenience in the way that a middle class person understands it is not what these folks are talking about. They may not have a car or a family member with one (or perhaps it is being used by a family member to get to work), public transportation may be unavailable, unreliable or inaccessible to them given their medical problems, and a large hospital ER is more likely to be on a bus route than a doctor's office. If they have jobs, they are usually not the kind that allow people to take a paid sick day to go to the doctor; they lose pay (and potentially their jobs). Despite efforts to have "extended hours", most ambulatory care offices are open mainly during regular business hours, during the day weekdays when the providers who work there want to work, not when it is necessarily most "convenient" for patients. Let's get this straight: it is not "convenient" to wait 6 hours in an ER to be seen; if this is better than the alternative, the alternative is seriously flawed.

Quality is another issue, and the quotation chosen is very open to criticism. The hospital had 4 days of complete control of the person's life, giving them their medicines and minimizing any external issues, while the doctor had 3 years in which the person was responsible for taking their medicine, choosing their diet, and deciding where to rank health among the many competing priorities in their lives. As any of us who have worked in medicine know, the control that was achieved in the hospital may well evaporate once someone returns to their regular environment.

In reality, this mostly comes down to money, to resources. The authors emphasize that not all the patients were uninsured, but among those who had insurance almost all had Medicaid. Not only is Medicaid not equivalent to private insurance (it pays less and lots of doctors do not take it), but it is only available to really poor people. People who are poor enough to have Medicaid have all those issues listed above under "Convenience" and "Cost" that go beyond the direct cost of medical care, and they inform every decision they make in their lives.

Policy, in almost every area, is made by the "haves", those with money and political power. While in some cases, at its rawest, the motivation can be "let's do for us, and screw those without power," it is usually more subtle, and done with much less intentionality, not to mention hostility. It is made from the perspective of people who have a lot, or at least a fair amount, and who cannot even imagine the lives, decisions, and trade-offs made every day by "have-nots." The "haves" may identify a lot that is wrong with the health care system, but they do not even think of things like not having transportation, or not being able to take off from work to go to clinics open during working hours, or not having child-care. They are not mean people, but they do not see.[10]

Who Pays the Most?

We also charge the poor more. Only people lacking insur-ance are billed the list prices for treatment, and the prices are often much higher (sometimes dozens of times higher) than what Medi-care or insurance companies pay because insurance companies al-ways negotiate significant discounts. In *Time Magazine,* Stephen Brill's article "Bitter Pill: Why Medical Bills are Killing Us"[11] cites case after case and example after example of how the current system of billing and reimbursement in health care and particu-larly in hospitals does this; it burdens the poor particularly. And yet no one escapes: it costs a fortune and is sapping the economy overall. Here are a few examples that he cites:

A troponin (blood test for a heart attack) test billed to an uninsured patient at $199. Medicare pays $14; a CBC (blood count) billed $157 when Medicare pays $11.
A nuclear heart scan for which Medicare pays $554 billed at $8,000.
A Medtronic spinal stimulator that lists for $19,000 from the manufacturer (if the hospital paid full list) billed to the patient for $49,000. [11]

As a personal example, a number of years ago I had outpa-tient surgery for a hernia repair. The hospital bill was $10,000. My insurance company at the time asked me to pay $400, they paid $1,600, and the hospital wrote off the remaining $8,000 as a "contractual adjustment." Had I been uninsured, I would have been billed the entire $10,000.

What was interesting to me in Brill's article is that most of the patients who received those outrageous bills were neither unemployed nor uninsured (although the one who was uninsured had the misfortune of being 64 rather than 65, so paid the $199 for her troponin instead of Medicare paying the $14). Rather, they were employed in low wage jobs and had low-quality insurance, with very low per-visit, per-year, or lifetime caps and were treated by the hospitals as if they were uninsured. One example: "'We don't take that kind of discount insurance' said the woman at MD Anderson [Cancer Center]" when a patient called to make an appointment; they needed to come up with $48,900 cash up front—and that was just the down payment! So, all estimates about the impact on the uninsured need to be augmented by understanding the impact on the *underinsured.*

Another example of health disparities can be found in relation to unintended pregnancies. Lawrence Finer and Mia Zolna looked at changes from 2001-2006, and found a slight increase in the rate: unwanted pregnancies as a percentage of all pregnancies rose from 48% to 49%. Women aged 15-17 had a small decrease but still had the highest rates. Otherwise, while the rates went down with increasing age, all groups 18 and up had a slight increase. But the important finding was the disparity in rates by factors other than age: by race/ethnicity, income, and educational level. The unintended pregnancy rate for women without a high school diploma (80 per 1,000) was more than 2.5 times that of college graduates (30); the rates for women who were high school grads and those with "some college" were in between. The rate for Black women (91) and Hispanic women (82) was also 2-3 times that of white non-Hispanic women (36). Income had the greatest disparity: the rate for women living below the poverty line (132) was more than 5 times the rate for women who lived above 200% of poverty.[12] These women do not necessarily get pregnant because they do not have health care, although access to contraception (especially what is called long-acting reversible contraception (LARC), such as IUDs that do not have to be used each time) can be limited with poor health care access. In any case, unintended pregnancy is a health issue that is tied to the social determinants of health.

So what is the result of this situation? Some poor people do not get access to appropriate care in a timely manner, and the overall cost to the system is higher for people getting care in the ER instead of an office. Worse, they are sometimes getting care in a hospital at a point in their illness when, if something still can be done, it is much more involved and expensive, further increasing costs.

This is ridiculous. It is not reasonable. But it is the way our system is designed. In the next chapter, we will look at another area, Primary Care, and how it can contribute to the health of the population—and is underused in the U.S.

References

1   Stillman M, Tailor M, Dead Man Walking, *N Engl J Med* October 23, 2013.

2. Preston J, Number of Illegal Immigrants in U.S. May Be on Rise Again, Estimates Say, *New York Times,* Sept 23, 2013.

3. Lowrey A, In Texarkana, uninsured and on the wrong side of a state line, *New York Times*, June 8, 2014.

4. http://www.dailykos.com/story/2007/07/10/356106/-Bush-today-on-health-care-just-go-to-an-emergency-room

5. Columbus Dispatch, http://www.dispatch.com/content/stories/local/2012/10/11/health-care-called-choice.html

6. Ibid #1

7. Tavernise, S. Cuts in hospital subsidies threaten safety-net care. *New York Times,* November 9, 2013.

8. Mian A, Sufi A, The financial vulnerability of Americans, House of Debt, April 7, 2014. http://houseofdebt.org/2014/04/07/the-financial-vulnerability-of-americans.html

9. Kangovi S, et al., Understanding why patients of low socioeconomic status prefer hospitals over ambulatory care , *Health Affairs* 32 (7): 1196-1203, July 2013

10. Ventres W, Gusoff G, Poverty Blindness: Exploring the Diagnosis and Treatment of an Epidemic Condition, *Journal of Health Care for the Poor and Underserved,* 25 (1): 52-62. February 2014

11. Brill S, Why medical bills are killing us, *Time,* April 4, 2013.

12. Finer LB and Zolna MR, Unintended pregnancy in the United States: incidence and disparities, 2006, *Contraception* 84(5):478-85, November, 2011

Chapter 5

Primary Care: The Essential Basis
For an Effective Healthcare System

The stone cold fact is that in the modern, industrialized world, the nations and regions that place a relatively greater emphasis on generalist medicine and primary care have consistently better health outcomes.[1]

—Jerry Kruse, M.D., executive associate dean
and CEO of Southern Illinois University Health Care

The last two chapters looked at the social determinants of health, making the case that it is in fact these characteristics of people's lives that make the biggest difference in their health, and that to have a healthy population we as a society need to invest in ensuring that all people have a fair chance of being healthy by having sufficient food, housing in safe places, and educational opportunity. All this is outside of what we usually think of as "healthcare." But even within the healthcare system itself our emphasis is misplaced, with much more money spent on the treatment of advanced disease (often too late) than on prevention and early diagnosis and treatment. This chapter will look at primary care, the cornerstone of any effective healthcare system. It will examine the contribution that primary care makes to the health of people and demonstrate how it is undervalued and undersupplied to Americans. We will look at what primary care is, who primary care providers are, why it is important, and the contributions that it makes to the health of people. We will also examine the shortage of primary care providers and what the implications of that shortage are.

Primary Care: The "Secret" to Good Healthcare

Primary care is the cornerstone of health care in most developed nations and in those less-developed nations with better health outcomes. In these countries, and in some regions within countries including within the U.S., the health system is built on a foundation of primary care, with the greatest resources spent on ensuring primary access, feeding into a smaller number of specialists, and costly hospital care at the top of the pyramid.

Most countries build their health systems on a foundation of primary care, as in Figure 5.1a. This is stable.

In the U.S., however, most of our emphasis is on specialists and hospitals, built on an inadequate primary care base, as in Figure 5.1b. This is unstable.

But is this necessarily a bad thing? While it may be true that this is the way that health care is organized in other countries, does this mean it is beneficial? Does the U.S., which is organized more like an upside-down pyramid, have a better solution? After all, we often hear that we have "the best health care in the world"! The data, however, belie that slogan. The U.S. may have the best "rescue care" (in the words of Donald Berwick, from the Institute for Healthcare Improvement and a former director of the Center for Medicaid and Medicare Services, CMS) for a particular need for a particular individual, but it scarcely has the best care for

Figure 5.1a

Health Systems Built on Primary Care

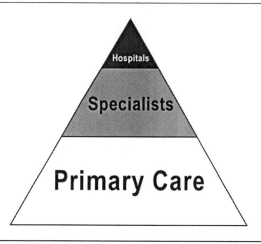

Figure 5.1b

Health Systems Based on Specialists and Hospitals

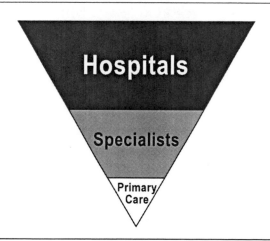

every condition for everyone. There are many people who do not have access to health care for financial reasons, and even those who do have access may get care that is not the "best" because our system is so skewed toward high-tech, high-cost interventions rather than those that lead to the best health outcomes—decreased mortality and better quality of life.

The "stone cold fact", as has been pointed out by family physician and health system leader Jerry Kruse, is that in the modern, industrialized world, the nations and regions that place a relatively greater emphasis on generalist medicine and primary care have consistently better health outcomes. Much of the research that supports this was developed by a group at the Johns Hopkins School of Public Health, led by the late Barbara Starfield. Among their many publications one of the most comprehensive is "Contribution of Primary Care to Health Systems and Health," published in the *Milbank Quarterly,* 2005.[1] They say:

Evidence of the health-promoting influence of primary care has been accumulating ever since researchers have been able to distinguish primary care from other aspects of the health services delivery system. This evidence shows that primary care helps prevent illness and death, regardless of whether the care is characterized by supply of primary care physicians, a relationship with a source of primary care, or the receipt of important features of primary care.

The evidence also shows that primary care (in contrast to specialty care) is associated with a *more equitable distribution of health in populations,* a finding that holds in both cross-national and within-national studies. The means by which primary care improves health have been identified, thus suggesting ways to improve overall health and reduce differences in health across major population subgroups.

The Johns Hopkins group identify several characteristics of health systems that have both better quality outcomes and lower cost:

- Distribution of health services equitably with respect to regional health care needs
- Universal or near-universal financial assistance guaranteed by a publicly accountable body
- Low or no co-pay for primary care health services
- Narrow range of physician incomes
- High percentage of physicians who are generalists (both with respect to the population and to all physicians)
- Relationship with a usual source of comprehensive, longitudinal medical care.

In Chapter 2, I provided evidence of the quality and cost rankings of different countries, particularly those "rich" countries in the OECD, and the poor performance of the U.S. in relation to these other countries in terms of population health outcomes. International comparisons also demonstrate that there is almost a linear relationship between the degree to which primary care is the basis of a nation's healthcare system (the "primary care score") and its rank in terms of quality health outcomes, as well as an inverse relationship with the cost of health care. That is, countries with a higher primary care score have better quality outcomes and lower cost. The U.S. primary care score and its health outcomes are both low, while its cost is high.

This relationship between primary care, cost, and outcomes also holds true within the U.S. Kathryn Baicker and Amitabh

Chandra looked at Medicare spending by state, and graphed it against quality measures (Figure 5.2).[3] There was an almost linear relationship, but in the opposite direction from which one would expect or hope: the states with the highest spending per beneficiary had the lowest quality indicators (based on standard measures, including such things as treatment after heart attack, heart failure, stroke, and pneumonia, use of influenza and pneumococcal immunizations, and end-of-life care).

Figure 5.2

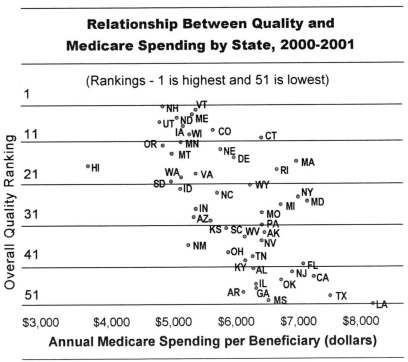

Relationship Between Quality and Medicare Spending by State, 2000-2001

Source: Baicker K and Chandra A, Medicare spending, the physician workforce, and beneficiaries' quality of care. *Health Affairs* 2004;W7:184-197.

Further analyzing these data, they compared both quality and cost to the ratio of both general practitioners and specialists per 10,000 residents, and found that as the ratio of specialists went up, the cost went up, but the quality went down; as the ratio of general practitioners per population went up, the opposite occurred: costs dropped and quality went up.

This is somewhat shocking in a nation that believes that "more is better" and that the best care comes from specialists (I use this term to describe non-primary care specialists). Clearly, when only the specialist is capable of providing what is necessary to improve a person's health, accessing that care is highly desirable. However, in settings such as in much of the U.S. (particularly in urban areas), where the ratio of specialists to primary care physicians (PCPs) is too great (as in the upside-down triangle pictured) there can be too much diagnostic testing and too many interventions. This not only increases the cost of care but increases the risk of harmful events occurring to the person being treated.

Specialists may be expert in their field, but are less knowledgeable about the differential diagnosis and preventive measures required in other areas. This is why studies have shown what, at first, seem to be contradictory findings: cardiologists are more likely than general internists to utilize appropriate preventive measures for heart disease (with family physicians in between), but PCPs are more likely to use the whole set of preventive measures recommended for a person. More important, specialists are likely to have greater suspicion that a disease with a set of symptoms is in their field, and to intervene using the tools at their disposal, even when the probability of the condition is low, for two reasons. One is that this is "what they do." Secondly, specialists have a fear of missing something that is in their area of expertise;

that fear is greater for them than it is for the primary care provider.

In short, added to the problem of those with fewer resources not getting necessary care, those who get more care may not be getting *better* care but rather more expensive care and more interventions. While occasionally part of the reason for this inversion is that some people, particularly those with good health insurance or lots of money, believe that "if some is good, more is better", and "if it costs more it must be better, and if it is better it is what I want", the fact is that it is doctors who order these tests, and they are primarily responsible for setting expectations for more and more expensive, high-tech care. The "more (or more expensive) is better" mentality may be valid, to some degree, for consumer items such as cars, appliances, houses, and jewelry. Unfortunately, those old saws are not true when it comes to health care. Frequently, less is better, and more is worse. This has increasingly been demonstrated with a number of ostensibly-preventive interventions that have been shown to both increase morbidity (because of false-positive tests that lead to dangerous but unnecessary intervention) and cost. Examples include PSA testing for prostate cancer (even the American Urological Association has come on board by not recommending this test for most men), mammography for breast cancer screening (for some populations), and the pelvic exam (the part where the provider puts hands inside, as distinct from the Pap smear screening test for cancer of the cervix) in asymptomatic women.

Many other studies have looked at U.S. communities and found consistently that higher primary care to specialist ratios have generated both higher quality and lower cost. In a widely-read *New Yorker* article, Atul Gawande compared the cost of care in the highest cost-per-person region of the country, the relatively low-income McAllen, TX, with the cost in a similarly lower income border community, El Paso, and found health outcomes not to be better despite the greater cost.[4] Thomas Bodenheimer and David West, discussing the low cost and high quality of care in the city of Grand Junction, CO, note 7 characteristics of the situation there that are responsible for these good results. They include:

> *...leadership by the primary care community; a payment system involving risk sharing by physicians; equalization of physician payment for the care of Medicare, Medicaid, and privately insured patients; regionalization of services into an orderly system of primary, secondary, and tertiary care; limits on the supply of expensive resources, including specialists, beds, and equipment; payment of primary care physicians for hospital visits; and robust end-of-life care.*[5]

More globally, Starfield and colleagues suggest that six mechanisms, "alone and in combination," provide the rationale for the beneficial impact of primary care on population health.

1. *greater access to needed services,*
2. *better quality of care,*
3. *a greater focus on prevention,*
4. *early management of health problems,*
5. *the cumulative effect of the main primary care delivery characteristics, and*
6. *the role of primary care in reducing unnecessary and potentially harmful specialist care.* [6]

The work of Starfield, Shi, Macinko, Baicker, Chandra and others, across regions and nations, that continues to show the benefit of primary care to the health of populations, as well as to individuals, has not, of course, been accepted by everyone. A number of health policy analysts have been critical of the data, even calling all these results "a statistical anomaly", which prompted Mark Ebell, a prominent family medicine researcher, to provide this definition of "statistical anomaly": "A consistent finding, in multiple nations and health systems, that disagrees with my current self-interest and bias." Besides being witty and accurate, it points to the two major motivators of such criticism: self-interest (mainly economic) and bias (based upon, again, self-interest, but this time more ego than money). Economic self-interest is easy to understand; if there are fewer high-tech procedures, then the specialists who do them could make less money, as might the hospitals in which they are provided.

Indeed, major restructuring of healthcare delivery in the U.S. is occurring and may result in making this dynamic worse. Many (and in some regions and specialties, most or all) medical practices are being bought up by hospitals or health systems (in the private, not national, sense of "system"; a group of hospitals and practice with common ownership). This takes advantage of a quirk in the Medicare payment structure, which is often emulated by private insurers. They pay more for procedures done in a hospital-owned setting than in a doctor's office, even if that setting *used to be* the doctor's office! The hospital makes more money and shares some of it with the doctors doing the procedures, protecting their income. The only downside is that Medicare—and by extension, all of us—lose by paying more for the same care.

Where Does Medical Care Actually Take Place?

In 1961, Kerr White published *The Ecology of Medical Care*[6], in which he analyzed the locations where medical care takes place. He found that in a community of 1,000 adults, in any given month about 750 would have symptoms of illness or injury, 250 would go to the doctor, 9 would end up in a hospital, and one would be hospitalized in an academic medical center. Forty years later, researchers at the Robert Graham Center repeated the study to identify changes that had occurred in the new millennium[7]. They found that care now occurs in a number of other locations, and that of that community of 1,000 adults, 65 saw a complementary or alternative medicine provider, 21 were seen in a hospital outpatient clinic, 14 received home healthcare, and 13 visited an emergency department. But the basic components of the ecology were little different: 800 had symptoms 217 saw a doctor (113 a primary care doctor), 8 were hospitalized, and less than 1 was in an academic medical center.

Primary care is a subset of ambulatory care. It is delivered by generalist providers, as opposed to specialists. The relationship between primary care providers (PCPs) and specialists is important, as is the ratio between the number of PCPs and the number of specialists in a community. The generalist can identify and care for most problems, and manages referrals to specialists when those are needed. The main reasons a generalist will refer a patient to a specialist are when a procedure (e.g., surgery) is needed that the primary care provider does not perform, when the illness that the patient has is either not apparent to the generalist after a reasonable workup or is not responding to usual therapy, when the therapy indicated for the condition is complex and ever-changing (as in chemotherapy for cancer), and when the disease identified is rare. Sometimes a PCP will refer to a specialist even when they are quite certain of the diagnosis and prognosis but, because the news is not good, refer to the specialist in hope that there may be something new in treatment, or at least to make sure that the patient has been given every opportunity to hear from the specialist that there is not.

What is the right ratio of PCPs to specialists? When there are enough specialists to provide the care that only they can deliver, and enough PCPs to deliver the care that they are capable of delivering, we have an appropriate balance between quality and cost. Most studies place the ideal ratio at about 50% primary care. In many parts of the U.S., however, including most major urban areas, the balance is way off; rather than demand driving supply, as in traditional economics, supply drives demand. Data demonstrate unequivocally that when there are more specialists there are more procedures, and in some cases there is clearly harm—certainly financial, and sometimes physical—to patients. This has been receiving ongoing coverage in the press, with such prominent articles as Steven Brill's major exposé in the February 2013 *Time* magazine *Bitter Pill: Why Medical Bills are Killing Us* mentioned earlier, and the remarkable ongoing series of articles in the *New York Times* by Elisabeth Rosenthal, including "Health Care's Road to Ruin"[9] and "Patients' Costs Skyrocket; Specialists' Incomes Soar."[10]

A major cause for the imbalance in reimbursement of PCPs and specialists can be traced to a committee convened by the American Medical Association (AMA), the Relative Value Scale Update Committee, called the RUC. Medicare payments are based on Relative Value Units (RVUs), which are assigned to virtually all physician activities (including procedures and physician visits), purporting to compare apples with oranges, office visits with heart surgery. Someone has to decide how many office visits are equivalent to heart surgery, especially when the size of the total pie that is being divided is fixed. That is the job of the Center for Medicare and Medicaid Services, but 95% of the time they take the advice of the RUC. And the composition of the RUC is dramatically skewed to specialists.

Members of this committee are supposed to operate free of self-interest, but the skew of values for different activities demonstrates that this cannot be so. In addition, RVUs are supposed to be assigned based on the amount of *work* involved, but for many things, especially procedures done by specialists, technological advances have made the amount of work and time required much less, while reimbursement has not similarly dropped. The time it takes to talk with and counsel a patient, however, has not changed with technological advances. Arguably, technology such as the Electronic Health Record (EHR) has increased it because of the time it takes to document unique patient interactions; specialists can be spared some of this by using text templates because of the similarity of their patient interactions. Given that reimbursement from most private insurers is based on multiples of Medicare rates, the decision about how Medicare reimburses affects virtually the entire third-party payment system. Over the last few years, several articles have appeared "exposing" the RUC and its practices, from the Kaiser Family Foundation[11], Princeton economist Uwe Reinhardt in his *New York Times* "Economix" blog,[12] and physician and Congressman Jim McDermott in the *New England Journal of Medicine*,[13] but so far its activities remain intact. The RUC is an interest group whose interests are skewed to specialists, but the decision is ultimately in the hands of Center For Medicare and Medicaid Services (CMS). Policy on reimbursement should not be based on in the input of interest groups, but on what is in the best interest of the people's health.

Bias is the other reason for such attitudes. Often subconscious, specialists may believe that because they *are* specialists, and because, in many cases they make so much more money (not all: for example, psychiatrists, many pediatric specialists, and many neurologists may have incomes similar to primary care physicians) they *must* be doing harder and more difficult work. To suggest otherwise creates serious cognitive dissonance. Primary care must be easier, because, well, it is paid less. The same "experts" who call studies demonstrating the benefit of primary care a "statistical anomaly" have also disparaged it, saying that there is no need for physicians to expend effort on uncomplicated primary care. On its face, there may be some validity to this; if the care is truly uncomplicated, it might well be delivered by non-physician (and even non-NP) providers, such as registered nurses (RNs).

Primary care improves the health of the population. It does this by relatively straightforward care, such as checking blood pressure and treating colds, but also through caring for people with multiple chronic diseases who need management of those conditions as well as coordination with whatever other specialists they are seeing. It improves the health of the population by providing preventive services, counseling and "asking for trouble" ("are you safe at home?"), discussing whatever other specialists may have recommended, and, of course, caring for acute complaints. This is hard, complex, time-consuming and difficult. Kimberly Yarnall and colleagues demonstrated that it would take 7.4 hours a day for a primary care physician to just provide the preventive services, not to mention all the other services above, especially chronic disease management.[14]

Carlos Moreno, chairman of the Department of Family Medicine at the University of Texas Health Science Center at Houston, states that "The question of what is intellectually challenging and worthy of training and intellect is a classic example of hubris perpetuated by specialists and academic health centers." He asks the following question of his medical students:

What is more intellectually challenging? Performing your 2000th knee arthroscopy? Performing your 3000th laparoscopic cholestectomy? Performing your 4,000th bronchoscopy? Performing your 5,000th colonoscopy? Performing your 6,000th intubation? Performing your 7,000th breast augmentation? Performing your 8,000th cataract removal? Reading your 10,000th MRI? Seeing your 15,000th case of acne?

Or:

Taking care of a 55 year-old with diabetes, hyperlipidemia, hypertension, coronary artery disease, chronic renal insufficiency, who is depressed, has a rash, erectile dysfunction, esophageal reflux and who is taking care of his elder mother with Alzheimer's dementia.[15]

In reviewing the charts of the patients seen by just one *first-year* family medicine resident in one clinic session, I noted she had seen (among others):

A woman with uncontrolled diabetes, recently discharged

from the hospital with diabetic ketoacidosis *[a serious life threatening complication]*;

A woman with anhedonia *[difficulty enjoying anything]* who feels "fat and alone"; she reports no "physical abuse"—her boyfriend "just" pushes her and she feels safe when she locks the door;

A woman for "well-woman exam" who came for Pap smear and prevention, with uncontrolled hypertension, very stressed from working her two jobs, having difficulty with her medication.

All had, in addition, other medical problems. This is uncomplicated primary care? The PCP has to deal with undifferentiated symptoms, with multiple chronic diseases, with balancing prevention with chronic and acute care, with ensuring that the social circumstances of the patient permit them to have a chance

Table 5.1

Comparison of the Work of Family Doctors and Specialists

Which is Harder?

SPECIALISTS	FAMILY DOCTORS
• Most patients already have diagnosis	• Sees undifferentiated patients
• Top 5 diagnoses 80%+ of practice	• Top 20 diagnoses <50% of practice
• Limited to one system, or less	• Multiple systems, multiple chronic diseases
• If problem outside their practice, refers	• If problem requires referral, also needs follow up
• Not interested in extraneous' issues	• "Asks for trouble"

of successfully managing their conditions, and inquiring about potential problems that the patient has not, for one reason or another, mentioned (as in "are you safe at home?"), which I call "asking for trouble." This issue should not be a competition, but the circumstances that reward specialists more than primary care doctors, leaving us with fewer PCPs, are in part based on inaccurate perceptions (Table 5.1). If we are to have a sufficient PCP to specialist ratio to provide the best possible care for Americans, it is important to challenge these biases.

The family physician must talk to her patients about obesity, but also about smoking. She must encourage the use of seat belts, but also bicycle helmets. She must be concerned about lead poisoning, but also about domestic violence.

The benefits of more primary care are so widely recognized that even multinational corporations like IBM can see the value. Several multi-national corporations, led by IBM, discovered that their health care costs were lower in many countries other than the U.S., and looked into why this was the case. It went far beyond the simple presence of a national health system, as it addressed the actual costs of care, not premiums. Their research indicated that the big differentiating factor was the presence of a strong primary care infrastructure, and they led the creation of the Patient-Centered Primary Care Collaborative (PCPCC), which now involves many corporations, health insurers, professional organizations and consumer groups interested in expanding the centrality of primary care in a patient-centered health system (www.pcpcc.org).

The Primary Care Conundrum

So we have a "primary care conundrum." We need more primary care providers, because health systems with the appropriate ratio of primary care to specialists have better health outcomes at the population and individual level, but we treat primary care doctors and other providers relatively poorly (especially with regard to income) compared to specialists and, at least in medical schools, may explicitly or implicitly discourage students from entering primary care. The payment gap between PCPs and many specialists has been growing for years. The ACA will increase payments to PCPs by 10%, but when PCP incomes may be only 1/3 of some specialists' incomes, it is not likely to make a very big difference.

Many arguments have been put forward, both in writing, in discussions with colleagues, and to students. They, include:

- It is not only primary care doctors that are relatively underpaid; so are many non-procedural specialists.
- There is not going to be an increase in the payment to physicians, so higher-paid specialists are going to have to take less money.
- It is not just about money; it is about lifestyle. Primary care doctors have to work too hard.
- It is not just about money; it is about status. Primary care doctors have lower status.
- It is not just about money; it is about intelligence. Primary care is just too easy.
- It is not just about money; it is about unrealistic expectations. Primary care is just too complex.

And on and on. These are not silly or spurious or even inaccurate statements, although the last two might be considered another "primary care conundrum", the one to which medical students are often subjected. All of these are things that family medicine and other primary care specialties have to think about, and address to the extent that it is within their control.

If we are to have a health care system that has the appropriate ratio of PCPs and specialists to maximize our population's health, income for PCPs, at least as a percentage of specialist income, is going to have to increase. The 20th Report of the Council on Graduate Medical Education (COGME)[16], a group formed by Congress to advise the Secretary of Health and Human Services, Senate Health Education Labor & Pensions Committee, and House Energy & Commerce Subcommittee on Health, contains a number of recommendations on how to achieve its goal of a minimum of 40% PCPs in the U.S. health system. These include payment policies that will achieve PCPs receiving at least 70% of median incomes of all other physicians, as well as a number of other recommendations related to medical education. It is a good recommendation, but real action from CMS will have to follow.

Who are Primary Care Providers?

Primary care can be delivered by several different physician specialties—family medicine (FM), general internal medicine (GIM), general pediatrics (GP)* but also by advanced registered nurse practitioners (NPs, or ARNPs) and physician's assistants (PAs) with generalist training. While these fields are not the

---

*There are limitations apparent in the use of the term "primary" care as the name for specialties that provide comprehensive, continuous care, which have led some to propose that other medical specialties, most commonly obstetrics/gynecology (OBG) and emergency medicine (EM), also are primary care. EM may be first contact care, but the care it provides is neither comprehensive nor continuous. OBGs are often the only provider women, especially younger women, see, but unless they are providing comprehensive care for those women and not just care for issues related to reproductive health, they do not meet the definition.

same, or interchangeable, they share several key features of primary care practice. These include first contact care, continuity of care, comprehensiveness of care, care based in the context of the patients' family and community. While these traits are characteristic of PCPs, the key feature that distinguishes them from other specialties is that they care for the whole person rather than a particular organ system, disease or procedure. For the primary care provider the relationship with their patient is based upon the relationship itself rather than on treatment of a particular condition. The patient is able to bring up *anything* to do with their health, or, indeed, their lives; the provider provides care for chronic diseases, acute problems that arise, and preventive care. The primary care provider works with the patient, and their family if the patient wishes, to manage all aspects of their care, to coordinate referrals to other providers, and to ensure that the recommendations of one provider do not contradict those of others.

To be sure, it is the character of the practice rather than the specialty certification that determines primary care. A physician trained in family medicine, the most generalist of specialties, can choose to limit their practice in a way that does not care for the whole person. The family physician or general internist who practices geriatrics is still providing primary care, but to a more narrowly-defined population; one who limits their practice to, say, skin conditions or sports medicine, is not providing primary care if they restrict their practice to that area, and do not also provide general comprehensive care.

On the other hand, a specialist may provide primary care to their patients if they extend it to the comprehensive management of acute and preventive issues as well as the specific disease for which they are seeing them. This is more common among pediatric specialists than those in adult medicine, for two reasons. First, the child with a chronic disease almost always has only one disease, (e.g., sickle cell anemia, type 1 diabetes, cystic fibrosis), so that, respectively, the pediatric hematologist, endocrinologist, or pulmonologist is usually the only specialist involved. Adults frequently have multiple chronic diseases—it is quite common for an adult to have, say, high blood pressure (hypertension), congestive heart failure, type 2 diabetes, arthritis, low thyroid, and depression. It is uncommon for one specialist to manage all of these conditions.

The second reason a specialist is more likely to provide primary care to a child than to an adult is that a child with a chronic disease is part of a family who is caring for them. The management of their disease, especially with young children, is done by their parents or adult caretakers. The child's chronic disease, in fact, may often be the focus of the entire family. This requires an understanding of family dynamics, including how this affects the child's siblings, and an ongoing relationship with those other family members, in a way that is different from what care for an adult requires. An adult cardiologist could, theoretically, provide all these services to a patient with heart disease, but generally prefers to work within their own subspecialty.

One suggestion frequently heard for "solving" the primary care crisis is to train more "mid-level" practitioners. Generally these are nurse practitioners (now called advanced registered nurse practitioners, or ARNPs, to include also nurse midwives and nurse anesthetists) and physician's assistants (PAs), but frequently also includes pharmacists and other health professionals. This was the theme of a lengthy editorial, "When the doctor is not needed," in the *New York Times* in December, 2012[17] It discusses how a variety of other health professionals can help to meet the health care needs of Americans when there are not enough physicians. In addition to pharmacists, nurse practitioners, and retail clinics (mostly staffed by nurse practitioners), the article identifies two other sources of care: "trusted community aides" and self-care. I will talk about these last two in a bit, but first would like to discuss the role of health professionals other than physicians to put these recommendations into context, and to provide a sense of what might reasonably be expected of them.

As the editorial points out, both pharmacists and nurse practitioners (and physician's assistants) have a significant knowledge base, and can (depending on state law) practice independently. Focusing on ARNPs, the American Association of Nurse Practitioners (AANP) lists on its website three levels of practice:[18]

Full Practice: State practice and licensure laws provide for nurse practitioners to evaluate patients, diagnose, order and interpret diagnostic tests, initiate and manage treatments—including prescribe medications—under the exclusive licensure authority of the of the state board of nursing. This is the model recommended by the Institute of Medicine and National Council of State Boards of Nursing.

Reduced Practice: State practice and licensure law reduce the ability of nurse practitioners to engage in at least one element of NP practice. State requires a regulated collaborative agreement with an outside health discipline in order for the NP to provide patient care.

Restricted Practice: State practice and licensure law restricts the ability of a nurse practitioner to engage in at least one element of NP practice. State requires supervision, delegation or team-management by an outside health discipline in order for the NP to provide patient care.

By these criteria, 17 states (mostly in the West plus DC) have full practice, 12 (mostly in the South) have restricted practice, and the rest (21) have reduced practice (widely distributed). The AANP and state nursing associations advocate for full practice, and, in general, medical societies (including those representing primary care, but this varies by state) have tended to oppose it. The arguments against "full scope" practice for ARNPs by medical organizations have focused on training, with an emphasis on the number of hours of education and training that they get compared to physicians before being licensed. In general, primary care organizations are supportive of ARNPs practicing, but want them to have "collaborative agreements" with physicians who supervise (in some manner) the care that they deliver, and can prevent them from performing activities for which they are not trained (e.g., doing surgery).

On the whole, I believe these to be invalid arguments for restricting ARNP practice. The best evidence for full ARNP practice is their performance in those 17 states (plus D.C.) where they do have full practice. There have not been significant reports of ARNPs practicing inappropriately, and they practice within their skill set and license, expanding care somewhat to the population. They are not unregulated or unlicensed; if their training has included doing minor surgery (e.g., removal of skin lesions, freezing warts, removing ingrown toenails) they may do that, just as primary care physicians do. They will not do, and will not be granted hospital privileges to do, major surgery, just as physicians who are not appropriately trained cannot.

ARNP and nursing organizations have also lobbied state legislatures to extend full practice privileges with the argument that this will help to address the shortage of primary care, especially in rural and underserved areas. This argument has likely had some validity, as it is in the sparsely populated rural Mountain and Western states where full practice is most common. It is very important to ensure that people everywhere have access to primary care, and there are large rural areas with insufficient numbers of providers. On a practical basis, however, there is no good evidence that ARNPs preferentially go to underserved, and in particular rural areas in significantly greater numbers than physicians do. This means that the licensing issue is an entirely separate one; just because ARNPs have a license to do full practice doesn't mean they will help solve the shortage of care given in rural areas.

Most ARNPs, and pharmacists, and other health professionals, want to stay in the cities and suburbs, just like their physician counterparts. They do not "diffuse" into underserved areas. Indeed, work by Robert Bowman indicates that of what he calls the 5 "forms" of primary care (family physicians, general internists, general pediatricians, nurse practitioners, and physician's assistants) only family physicians distribute in proportion to the population. That is, about 20% of people live in rural areas and about 20% of FPs practice there.[19] The retail clinics at which many ARNPs work, often based in chain pharmacies, are mostly located in cities and suburbs, where their owners can make more money, and serve basically the same population that more traditional medical practices do. While not all health profession students who are from rural areas will return to them, they are far more likely to move there than those from urban and suburban communities. In the next chapter, I make the case for prioritizing training medical students who come from rural areas for this reason, and the same applies to other health professionals. If a nurse from a rural community, who has family and roots there, is trained to be an ARNP, s/he is likely to return. If most ARNPs are from the suburbs, they are unlikely to move to a rural area.

The licensing issue, as noted above, is separate. If ARNPs are qualified to practice independently, as I believe they should be, they should have this scope of practice. If they are not, it would be inappropriate to grant practice privileges only in those areas where there are no physicians; in essence, that second class care is OK for some people. This is an issue to which primary care physicians should be exquisitely sensitive, since they have faced the same argument. It has been suggested that family physicians should be able to have a full scope of practice (obstetrics, sometimes surgical obstetrics, neonatal care, endoscopy, fracture care, etc.) only in areas where there are no specialists who make their living doing these things. The argument in both cases is more about restraint of trade than quality.

Of course, not all ARNPs (and even fewer PAs) enter primary care practice. While much of the emphasis has been on the use of professionals other than physicians to provide primary care, many ARNPs and PAs work for specialists, in large hospitals, and in metropolitan areas. We do not hear of a shortage in these fields mainly because there is none. A big part of the reason that they work in urban/suburban settings is that, as noted above, like physicians, they are predominantly from these areas and can make more money in these roles, as do the physicians who employ them. Another reason why they don't fan out into rural areas is that many ARNPs were hospital nurses prior to receiving advanced training, and it is natural and comfortable for them to continue in the same setting, focusing on the area (heart disease, kidney disease, cancer, intensive care, surgical specialties) that they are familiar with. PAs, possibly because their training does not include a nursing background, are very commonly attracted to positions in the emergency room and as surgical assistants.

Finally, two dynamics that are rarely understood exacerbate the primary care shortage: ARNPs choose specialty care because of work conditions and pay. On the work conditions front, to the extent that some specialties also have more regular work hours and a limited scope of work, they may seem more attractive. The limited scope of work (which is not to say less work or less difficult work) can make them appealing. The stereotype is that specialists see difficult problems while primary care providers see mostly colds and blood pressure checks. But this is not the case. Primary care is complex, as it sees both undifferentiated patients and those with multiple chronic diseases. Most specialty care is more routine, seeing a much more limited set of diagnoses with a more limited set of interventions; the typical specialist will see a much narrower range of diagnoses than a family doctor. An ARNP, particularly if they are a former hospital nurse and not trained specifically as a Family Nurse Practitioner, can be an in-depth expert in this limited range of diagnoses, following people with congestive heart failure for cardiologists or those with diabetes for endocrinologists, managing chemotherapy recipients for oncologists, using algorithms to care for people in intensive care units, doing pre- and post-operative care for orthopedists and other surgeons. They are not called upon to go outside of the set of diagnoses and treatment options with which they are familiar; following the model of the physicians with whom they work, when a patient's problem is not in their narrow area, it is referred elsewhere. This means, however, that ARNPs who work in these settings have no positive impact addressing the shortage of primary care.

The targeted but limited expertise of such nurse specialists explains why they function so well clinically in subspecialties. It works well financially because the doctors (or hospitals, or health systems) that employ them are reimbursed at specialist physician rates (already very high) for work that is done by others. Thus they can afford to pay such "physician extenders" relatively well compared to folks working in primary care. Reimbursement for "teams" follows the model of reimbursement for physicians: care for a limited set of diagnoses in a detailed way, especially when it involves procedures, is paid much better than management of complex sets of interactive diagnoses.

ARNPs, then, are making a rational choice: more money and better working conditions. Primary care practice is challenging because the same patient often has multiple conditions, and interventions that help one may make another worse. While efforts to build teams, and have each professional work at the "top of their license", is important, so is payment. As long as primary care is reimbursed at lower rates it will continue to face challenges in recruitment of physicians, nurses, and other team members.

The reality is that there are not enough primary care providers even if we count the ARNPs and PAs in primary care. (Tables 5.2 and 5.3) In 2010, there were 222,000 primary care doctors (family physicians, general practitioners, general internists, general pediatricians and geriatricians), or one for every 1,358 people, and an additional 86,000 primary care NPs and PAs, for a total of 308,000, or one primary care provider for every 1,000 people. This overall ratio is good, but the geographic distribution is not. In some areas coverage is very good, with a provider to patient ratio of 1:500. In others, it is terrible, with a ratio of 1:5,000 in various Primary Care Service Areas (PCSAs).

There are about 5,000 PCSAs with a deficit, which are short about 54,000 PCPs. This is about the same as the excess of PCPs

Table 5.2

Number of Primary Care Physicians, 2010

Specialty	# of providers (2010, adjusted*)	% time spent in Primary Care	# of PCPs adjusted for % PC time
Family Docs	89,066	0.95	84,613
GPs	9,870	1	9,857
Internists	95,533	0.8	76,697
Pediatrics	50,258	0.95	47,745
Geriatrics	3,575	0.95	3,396
Total	248,302		222,308

* Adjusted for physicians retired or otherwise out of primary care.

Table 5.3

PAs and ARNPs in Primary Care

	Total	% Primary Care
PAs	70,383	43%
NPs	106,073	52%

in the 1,600 PCSAs with a surplus. Unsurprisingly, the PCSAs with deficits are in the rural parts of the U.S. that make up the vast majority of our land mass. This work, by the Robert Graham Center of the American Academy of Family Physicians, demonstrates a need for an additional 50,000-60,000 more PCPs by the year 2025 to accommodate population growth and aging as well as expansion of coverage to more people as a result of the Affordable Care Act (ACA).[20] We have to have strategies to meet that need. Optimism may not be justified. There are more applicants to primary care positions, but most of those who will actually practice primary care, even more in those rural PCSAs, are going to be family physicians. Several studies continue to show decreased interest in primary care among internal medicine residency graduates, with about 80% pursuing subspecialty training and a majority of the remainder practicing as hospitalists.[21,22]

In addition, there is the issue of money and health insurance. Many people, particularly the working poor, whether in cities or rural communities, will continue to lack health insurance even after the ACA is fully operational, especially if they live in a state which has not expanded Medicaid. And while some may have the cash to go to a retail clinic, if one is available, most are unlikely to have enough to cover a big ER or hospital bill. Plus, even where Medicaid is expanded, not all providers take Medicaid. This means that people will continue to lack access to care because of geographic and financial barriers. And if they can get seen for primary care, maybe through a retail clinic, maybe via a nurse practitioner or primary care doctor, specialist care is becoming increasingly unavailable to Medicaid (and, of course, to uninsured) patients. This has been documented in several articles in the *Los Angeles Times*[23] and the *New York Times.*[24]

While there have been enough specialists for Medicare, if not Medicaid, even this may be changing, as many hospitals also see Medicare as a poor payer. As physician practices continue to be acquired by hospitals, the cost of care is increasing.[25] And because pharmacists, PAs and ARNPs are even more likely than physicians to be employed by big hospitals or health system or other corporations (such as the chain pharmacies in which most pharmacists work and which host most retail clinics), they will not solve the problem.

There are some solutions, however. The *New York Times* editorial cited earlier above also discusses the use of non-traditional health workers, which it calls "trusted community aides." While it refers to two pediatric practices where patients pay about $17 a visit, this concept is in much wider use—and should be used even more. Sometimes called community health workers or (from the Spanish) *promotores* (health promoters), these are lay people who have been trained to do basic health assessments, recommend treatment (usually in consultation with a nurse or doctor by phone) and help patients do a better job of taking care of their own health. They are most effective when they are from the community and culture of the patients for whom they care. Because they are recruited from the communities where they will serve, and in which they have roots and ties, they are highly likely to continue to serve those communities. This model has worked for dental care in Alaskan Native communities, and in urban inner city communities like Camden, New Jersey[26]. In the case of rural communities, the concept can also be used to increase the skills of nurses. Enhancing and expanding the training of a nurse in a rural community, of someone who has family there, or training community health workers who live there, will improve access in those areas in a way that simply will not happen by producing more doctors and nurse practitioners who come from and train in major urban centers.

The last suggestion in the *Times* editorial is for self-care. This is absolutely critical, and can be used for many of the diagnoses (notably excluding immunizations) that retail clinics provide care for. For colds, for minor injuries, people should be able to care for themselves. Where it gets tricky is when the "self" has multiple chronic diseases (say diabetes, hypertension, congestive heart failure, chronic lung disease, arthritis, low thyroid, and high cholesterol—a very common combination in any primary care practice). These people can provide more of their own care, but still need the guidance of a skilled health professional, most often a primary care physician.

In sum, all of these ideas have merit, but the issue of geographic and socioeconomic diffusion is largely ignored by most of those who tout their profession as the solution. As health policy expert Don McCanne notes about the problem of specialists not seeing poor people, "If we had an improved Medicare single payer system that treated everyone equitably, we would not have this problem."[27]

Yes, certainly there would still be problems, but that would be a great start.

It can be done. Some years ago, Canada confronted a sharp drop in students choosing family medicine, their main primary care specialty. Policies put in place in their medical schools and especially in reimbursement for family physicians, dramatically reversed this trend in just a few years.[28] Policies that address the real problem can be effective. Everyone—doctors, nurses, nurse practitioners, pharmacists, physician's assistant, et al—will have to work "at the top of their license" so that doctors are not expected to "do it all" and the others have the opportunity to really demonstrate their skills. It is, however, mainly an issue of public policy, not individual choice. Our government, through Medicare and Medicaid (and other insurers will follow suit) need to develop a plan for making the reimbursement for primary care more equitable.

References

1   Kruse, J. Personal communication

2   Starfield B, Shi L, Macinko J, Contribution of Primary Care to Health Systems and Health, *Milbank Quarterly* ;83(3):457-502, 2005

3   Baicker K and Chandra A, Medicare spending, the physician workforce, and beneficiaries' quality of care. *Health Affairs* 2004;W7:184-197.

4   Gawande, A, The cost conundrum, *New Yorker,* June 1, 2009.

5   Bodenheimer T, West D, Low-cost lessons from Grand Junction, Colorado, *N Engl J Med* 363(15):1391-3, October, 2010.

6   Ibid # 2

7   White KL, Williams TF, Greenberg BG. The ecology of medical care. *N Engl J Med*; 265:885–892, 1961.

8   Green, LA et al., The ecology of medical care revisited, *N Engl J Med*; 344:2021-2025, June 28, 2001.

9   Rosenthal E, Health Care's Road to Ruin, *New York Times*, December 21, 2013.

10   Rosenthal E, Patients' costs skyrocket, specialists incomes soar, *New York Times*, January 18, 2014.

11   Klepper B and Kibbe DC, Quit the RUC, *Kaiser Health News*, Jan 20, 2011.

12   Reinhardt U, The Little-Known Decision-Makers for Medicare Physicians Fees, *New York Times,* Dec 10, 2010

13   McDermott J, Harnessing Our Opportunity to Make Primary Care Sustainable, *N Engl J Med;* 364:395-397, February 3, 2011.

14   Yarnall KS, Pollak KI, Ostbye T, et al. Primary care: is there enough time for prevention?, *Am J Pub Health* 93(4):635-41, April, 2003.

15   Moreno, C, Personal Communication

16   Council on Graduate Medical Education, 20th Report, December 2010.

17   When the doctor is not needed, Editorial, *New York Times,* December 16, 2012.

18   American Association of Nurse Practitioners, http://www.aanp.org/legislation-regulation/state-legislation-regulation/state-practice-environment, accessed March 31, 2014.

19   Bowman RC, They really do go, *Rural and Remote Health 8: 1035. (Online), 2008.*

20   Petterson SM, et al., Unequal Distribution of the U.S. Primary Care Workforce, *Amer*

Fam Phys 87(11):1, June 1, 2013.

21 Garibaldi, RA, Popkave C, Bylsma W, Career plans for trainees in internal medicine residency programs, *Acad Med* 80(5):507-12, May 2005

22 Hauer KE, Durning SJ, Kernan WN et al., Factors associated with medical students' career choices regarding internal medicine. *JAMA* 300(10):1154-64, 2008.

23 Gorman A, *Los Angeles Times,* December 15, 2012 Health care crisis: not enough specialists for the poor, and February 25, 2013, Healthcare overhaul may threaten California's safety net."

24 Pear R, States Can Cut Back on Medicaid Payments, Administration Says, *New York Times,* February 25, 2013

25 Alexander A, Garloch K, Raynor D, As doctors flock to hospitals, bills spike for patients, *Charlotte Observer*, December 17, 2012

26 Gawande A, The Hot Spotters: can we lower medical costs by giving the neediest patients better care?, *New Yorker,* January 24, 2011.

27 McCanne, D., Quote-Of-The-Day, Dec 7, 2012. www.pnhp.org/news/quote-of-the-day

28 Rosser WW, Colwill JM, Kasperski JK, et all, Patient-Centered Medical Homes in Ontario, *N Engl J Med*; 362:e7 January 21, 2010

Chapter 6

The Role of Medical Education in
Perpetuating the Health System

Medical schools...are the only institutions in our society that can produce physicians.

—Fitzhugh Mullan et al.[1]

Doctors have to go to medical school. They have to learn their craft, master skills, and gain an enormous amount of knowledge. They also, and this is at least as important, need to learn how to think and how to solve problems. They need to learn how to be life-long learners because new knowledge is constantly being discovered, and old truths are being debunked. Therefore, they must learn to un-learn, and not to stay attached to what they once knew to be true yet no longer is. They also need, in the face of drinking from this fire-hose of new information and new skills, to retain their core humanity and their caring, the reasons that, hopefully, most of them went into medicine. Is medical school currently doing a good job of producing the doctors that this country needs? Are they learning the skills that they need to be competent, and compassionate? Has medical education changed as our needs have changed?

This chapter will look at medical school education, its strengths and weaknesses, at who gets selected for medical school, and what they learn. Medical school comes first in doctors' careers. It shapes their attitudes toward medicine and is where they make the decision about what specialty they will enter. In the fol-

125

lowing chapter, we will discuss residency training, where medical school graduates really learn the clinical specialties that they will practice.

The majority of medical schools, and those with the large majority of medical students, are allopathic schools, those that give an M.D. degree, as opposed to osteopathic schools, which give the D.O. Most of these allopathic schools are part of an "academic health center" (AHC), which means, at a minimum, that they are combined with a teaching hospital. In addition, most have large biomedical research enterprises, which depend largely on many Ph.D. faculty who are, if they are good and lucky, externally funded by the National Institutes of Health (NIH), or other smaller federal and private agencies and organizations. Some or many of them spend some of their time teaching the "basic sciences" (biochemistry, anatomy, physiology, microbiology, pharmacology, pathology) to medical students.

This history goes back 100 years, to the Flexner Report of 1910[2]. After establishing the Council on Medical Education in 1904, the American Medical Association (AMA) asked the Carnegie Foundation to evaluate medical schools. Carnegie hired educator Abraham Flexner to examine and evaluate the multitude of medical schools that existed at the time. Flexner recommended closing many, some of which were little more than for-profit apprenticeship programs without a scientific basis. He also recommended that medical schools be based upon the model of Johns Hopkins: part of a university (from the German tradition), grounded in science, and built upon a core curriculum in the biological sciences. This has been the model ever since.

One hundred years later, these medical schools and the AHCs of which they are a part have grown to enormous size, concentrating huge basic research facilities (Johns Hopkins alone receives over $300 million a year in NIH grants) and tertiary and quaternary medical services—high tech, high complexity treatment for rare diseases or complex manifestations of more common ones. They have often lost their focus on the health of the actual community of which they are a part. So are they still the best places to teach medical students?

The fact is that most doctors who graduate from medical school will not practice in a tertiary-care AHC, but rather in the community. As discussed in the last chapter, a disproportionate number of them will choose specialties that are of little or no use in many communities that need doctors. Many students will, if they can (i.e., if their grades are high enough) choose subspecialties that can only be practiced in the high-tech setting of the AHC or the other relatively small number of very large metropolitan hospitals, often those with large residency training programs. As these students look around at the institution in which they are being educated, the AHC, they see an enormously skewed mix of specialties. For example, 10% of doctors may be anesthesiologists, and there well may be more cardiologists than general internists. While this is not the mix in the world of practice, and still less the mix that we need to have for an effectively functioning health system, it is the world in which they are being trained.

The extremely distorted mix of medical specialties in the AHC is not necessarily "wrong", as it reflects the atypical mix of patients who are hospitalized there. It is, however, a mix that can lead students to have a very skewed idea of what conditions a set of symptoms is likely to represent, and what the appropriate treatments might be. Most of what people present with in the community is taken care of by PCPs, or by referral to community-based specialists. It is the unusual conditions that get referred to the AHC.

Recall the "ecology of medical care" model, developed first by Kerr White in 1961[3] and replicated by the Robert Graham Center of the American Academy of Family Physicians in 2003, as discussed in the last chapter. Figure 6.1 shows what happens to the health care needs of 1,000 people in a community. 800 may not feel well in a given month, but only ¼ of these see a doctor, 8 are admitted to the hospital, and less than 1 is admitted to an academic medical center. Thus, the population that students mostly learn on is atypical, heavily skewed to the uncommon. It is not representative of even all hospitalized people, not to mention the non-hospitalized ill (and still less the healthy-but-needing-preventive care) in the community.[4]

Figure 6.1

The Ecology of Medical Care: Where Medical Care Takes Place in the Community

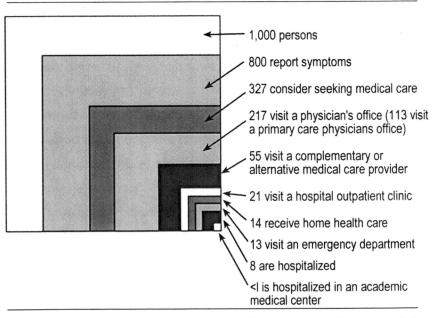

- 1,000 persons
- 800 report symptoms
- 327 consider seeking medical care
- 217 visit a physician's office (113 visit a primary care physicians office)
- 55 visit a complementary or alternative medical care provider
- 21 visit a hospital outpatient clinic
- 14 receive home health care
- 13 visit an emergency department
- 8 are hospitalized
- <1 is hospitalized in an academic medical center

Source: Reprinted with permission from Green, LA et al. The ecology of medical care revisited, *N Engl J Med* 344: 2021-2025, 2001.

So why do we continue to educate medical students in the rarefied setting of the AHC? Is this really the best place to train physicians? What are the incentives for schools to continue this structure? What other ways might they be organized? How would that benefit society? Is change possible?[5]

In order to answer these questions, it is a good idea to look at the incentives that medical schools have to maintain the current situation. This includes understanding how they are "ranked" and what those leading them perceive to be of greatest importance.

How Medical Schools are Ranked: Consumers Report-type Evaluations or James Bond-like brand-name dropping?

Often it appears that Americans are obsessed by "rankings", about knowing what is "the best." Sometimes, in the case of consumer products, we have ratings organizations like Consumers Union that have explicitly-stated criteria for why they say which is the best car, TV, stereo, or video game. They also will indicate what they believe to be the best value in order to help us decide if we want to spend a lot more money on a product whose performance is only marginally better. However, in ranking universities, and in particular medical schools, the criteria are often much less explicit, more subtle, and more subjective. The best-known rankings of colleges, universities, and graduate schools in a wide variety of areas, including medicine, are those of *U.S. News and World Report*.

In his book *David and Goliath*[6], Malcolm Gladwell has a chapter in which he discusses student success, and how different institutions have different strengths which benefit different types of students; there is not one "best" ("If I'd gone to the University of Maryland, I'd still be in science"). The same is true for medical schools. A reasonable question, both for a potential immediate consumer (a future student) and a future consumer of the products produced by the school (in the case of medical school, health care provided by its graduates) would be "what do the rankings mean?" How are they derived? What do they reflect about the "product" being evaluated? What criteria are they using? Are these criteria that accurately assess what I am looking for in a school? Are these down-to-earth, utilitarian, *Consumers Report*-type evaluations or are they more like James Bond-style brand-name dropping? Of course, if what one is looking for in a school is indeed cachet—its status, fame and brand-name recognition—then there is no difference. If, however, one is looking for outcomes—what is the success of that school in educating people in the area in which I wish to be educated, or how well that school does in producing the doctors America needs, it is important to look at the criteria being used and the degree to which they accurately predict outcomes.

In general, most educators do not feel that *U.S. News* rankings accurately reflect what they purport to be ranking—the quality of a school in a particular area. These criticisms probably are more vocal from those who believe that they are ranked lower than they should be, but even those ranked highly will usually acknowledge, *sotto voce*, that they are not completely accurate—although they are pleased to be ranked highly. Probably in response to ongoing criticism from the higher education community, *U.S. News* has begun to publish the criteria it uses for ranking, the weight that they give to each criterion, and the method that they use to gather the information. This helps us to assess the validity of those criteria. (*Validity* is a concept that is used in research to evaluate the quality of a tool being used; it is the degree to which it actually measures what it supposed to be measuring.)

Medical schools are comprehensively ranked by *U.S. News* for their quality of <u>Research</u> and <u>Primary Care</u>. For Research the criteria include peer assessment, selectivity (how high were the pre-admission grades and scores on the Medical College Admissions Test (MCAT) of its students, and the percent of applicants accepted—lower is 'better'), faculty:student ratio, number and dollar amount of research grants. For Primary Care, peer assessment and selectivity are again considered but rather than measuring research grants, they look at the total number (#) and percentage (%) of graduates entering primary care residency training. In addition, *U.S. News* reports top-ranked schools in a variety of program areas (AIDS, Family Medicine, Geriatrics, Internal Medicine, Pediatrics, Rural Health, Women's Health), but in these areas the rankings are done *entirely* by peer assessment. Because of the importance of primary care as a determinant of population health, I will focus upon the Primary Care and Family Medicine rankings, because they are not necessarily associated with the schools that are doing the best jobs of producing primary care or family physicians.

Peer assessment counts for about 40% of the weight of the rankings for Primary Care. Deans of medical schools, department chairs in the "primary care" specialties, and directors of residencies in those primary care specialties are asked to list the top schools, in their opinion. These are then added and weighted. Selectivity accounts for about 15%, faculty-student ratio another 15%, and these are the same as measured for Research. The final 30% consists of the schools' self-report of the percent of students graduating who enter the primary care specialties, defined by *U.S. News* as family medicine, general internal medicine, and general pediatrics.[7]

Because a student interested in primary care or family medicine might choose a school that is highly ranked in those areas, it is of value if the highly-ranked schools are indeed strong in those areas. Let us deconstruct those three sets of criteria. One important criterion, perhaps the most important and objective is the percent of students actually entering the primary care specialties, yet there are some problems in the data. What is, for example, the definition of entering a "general internal medicine" residency? Virtually all schools count everyone entering an internal medicine residency as primary care. The problem is that after completing that residency a very large percentage enter subspecialty training (to become cardiologists, gastroenterologists, endocrinologists, etc.) and never practice primary care. In recent years the percent of internal medicine residency graduates entering subspecialty fellowships on completing their residencies has been increasing so much that the number of students entering internal medicine residencies who actually become primary care/general internists is becoming vanishingly small.[8,9]

So a school with a high primary care ranking because a large percent of its graduates enter internal medicine may in fact be producing very few primary care doctors. Moreover, if schools that are in fact producing very low numbers of practicing primary care physicians can still receive high rankings for primary care, they have little incentive to change their programs to help produce more PCPs and begin to address the current shortage.

Arguably, the most sensitive indicator of primary care production by a school is entry into family medicine, because virtually all family medicine residents become primary care doctors. Thus, when the number of students entering family medicine is up, it means that interest in primary care is up, and it is likely that the percent of students entering internal medicine who will become general internists is also up. When the number entering family medicine is down, so is the number of internists entering general internal medicine. Ironically, however, the Family Medicine ranking of a school does not take this into account; as noted above, for Family Medicine (as well as a number of other areas), the sole ranking criterion is Peer Assessment. This would be fine if this criterion identified the schools producing the most family physicians; it would help identify them for prospective students.

Peer Assessment, however, also has its flaws. These include: people's memories are dated (they may remember that a place was good and so assume it still is), they may assume that a place that is good in many things is good in everything (e.g., Harvard gets votes for great family medicine, even though they have no family medicine department), and the ratings, especially from deans and chairs, may reflect the prominence of the faculty in primary care rather than the school's success in producing primary care physicians. Finally, because the chairs and residency directors surveyed are from all three specialties, the degree to which one or more of them is particularly strong or weak (or perceived as particularly strong or weak) can color the assessment. Below we will look at objective data (what percent of a school's graduates enter family medicine) and compare it to the results obtained by "peer assessment."

Selectivity is an ironic criterion as a measure of quality in Primary Care. The fact is that the more selective a school is, the lower the primary care production. This is, in brief, because students from families in relatively upper class suburbs who went to excellent prep schools (public or private) and thus are likely to have the highest grades are also the least likely to enter primary care. Students from rural and inner-city areas, as well as those from minority and lower income backgrounds are more likely to enter primary care, but are also less likely to have the highest grades. Their grades are lower because they have less elite preparation, not because they are less smart or less capable and certainly not because they will be inferior doctors. Finally, while the idea of a *high faculty-student ratio* sounds good, it probably doesn't matter to students unless those faculty members are actually teaching. In fact, schools with higher faculty-student ratios don't usually have more teachers; the additional faculty are either doing research (good for the research criterion, less obviously so for primary care) or providing clinical care in a variety of settings that have little or nothing to do with educating students.

Is there a correlation between high *U.S. News* Primary Care rankings and entry of students into primary care? It isn't a strong one, as can be seen in Table 6.1, which compares *U.S. News's* Top 50 for Primary Care and Top 10 for Family Medicine with those schools that actually produced the highest raw number and percent of students entering family medicine residencies in 2009.

More important, none of the criteria that *U.S. News* uses for its overall ranking of medical schools takes into account any characteristic that would indicate whether it is doing a good job of serving society, of producing physicians who want to (based on their entry characteristics), can (by virtue of their training and specialty choice) and do (based on their practice type and location) meet the unmet healthcare needs of the U.S. In addition to its poor portrayal of the primary care quality of a school, these criteria include no consideration of their efforts to address health inequities or increase the level of justice within our society.

Table 6.1

Comparison of Top Primary Care Schools
and Actual Production of Primary Care Physicians

Of the U.S. News "Top 50" in Primary Care:

- Only ten were among the "Top 15" in either percent or total number of students entering family medicine.

- Fully half (26) of these "Top 50" primary care schools were below the national average of 8.2% of students entering family medicine. Thirteen had five or fewer students entering family medicine and seven had two, one or zero!

- Conversely, only six of the top fifteen schools in % of students entering family medicine, and only nine of the top sixteen schools ranked by number of students entering family medicine, made *U.S. News's* "Top 50" for primary care.

Of the *U.S. News* "Top 10" for family medicine ranked only by peer assessment:

- Only three were in the "Top 15" entering family medicine by %, and three by total number of students entering family medicine residencies. Two schools were both. So a total of four *U.S. News's* "Top 10" medicine schools for family medicine were actually in the "Top 15" in either category. And of these four, the highest rank for % of students was # 11, and for total number, the highest rank was # 4.

- Among that group of "Top 10" family medicine schools, three (30%) were far below the national average for percent of students entering family medicine: seven students (4.1%); six students (4%) and two students (2.2%)!

- Conversely, only three of the top fifteen schools by number of students, and only four of the "Top 15" by percent of students entering family medicine residencies made *U.S. News's* "Family Medicine Top 10."

Source: Freeman J, Delzell J, Medical school graduates entering family medicine: increasing overall number. *Fam Med* 44(9):613-614, 2012.

The Social Mission of Medical Schools

Frustration with this *U.S. News*-type rating system led researchers from the Medical Education Futures Study (MEFS) at George Washington University and collaborators to develop and publish a different method of ranking medical schools, by social mission.[7] It challenges the notion that "good" medical schools are "good" at everything. It evaluates different outcomes, in particular the degree to which medical schools meet their "social mission", or to put it another way, the degree to which they produce the physicians who will take care of the American people. More to the point, since it can be argued that most medical school graduates take care of some American people, they measure the degree to which a school produces physicians who will take care of those people who need care the most because they don't already have doctors. This means largely those in poor communities, rural communities, and minority communities (and especially those communities that overlap as two or three of these). The researchers looked at three characteristics of graduates:

- What percent of their graduates are practicing primary care?
- What percent of their graduates are practicing in designated Health Professions Shortage Areas (HPSAs)? and...
- What percent of their graduates are members of underrepresented minority groups?

These may not be comprehensive measures of a medical school's social mission, but they are pretty straightforward, and are far better at trying to measure social impact than any other ranking system in use.[10]

In their actual rankings, the MEFS researchers took two

other steps to try and ensure that this is an accurate portrayal of the actual situation. The first is that they examined students in the graduating classes of 1999-2001, and looked at them 8 years after graduation, after they had completed residency and perhaps subspecialty fellowship training. This allowed them to get a much more accurate picture of who is actually practicing primary care. Similarly, it also means that those who are practicing in HPSAs have been doing it for several years, not just for one or two. The results showed that, overall, public schools did much better than private schools, and Southern, Midwestern, and Western schools did better than Northeastern schools.

In an effort to equitably assess a school's percent of under-represented minority students, the actual percent of underrepresented minority graduates was compared to the percent of the underrepresented minority population for the state for public medical schools, and the national percentage of underrepresented minorities (26.5%) for private schools, which are presumed to draw from a more national base. Thus, for example, the University of Iowa has a positive ratio with 8.1% minority students in a state that is only 6% minority, while the *Universidad de Puerto Rico en Ponce* has a negative ratio because, even though their students are 82.5% underrepresented minorities, their "state" is 98.8%.

The underrepresented minority scores for the 3 historically black medical schools, Morehouse, Meharry and Howard are so high, compared to the national average (they are all private) that they are easily the top 3 in the overall social mission score. This tends to wash out the significant differences between them in the other two areas. For example Meharry does well in producing physicians who actually practice primary care (49.3%) compared to Howard (36.5%). Howard, however, does better at placing students in Health Professional Service Areas (HPSAs) (33.7%) than Meharry (28.1%). Ponce, despite its negative underrepresented minority score, and also a negative primary care physician score, ranks #9 nationally in total social mission score. This is based on its high rate of physicians practicing in HPSAs, because so much of its service area in Puerto Rico is in HPSAs.

The data can be analyzed in a number of ways. Osteopathic schools have a much higher rate of producing primary care doctors, but none were in the top 20 because their percent of underrepresented minorities are low. A few top NIH research schools (4, to be exact) "defied the trend" and were in, at least, the top quartile of social mission scores, again all public schools. Other than the historically black schools, private schools were nowhere to be seen. This is presumably because public schools which are supported by their states identify at least part of their mission as supplying the doctors that the state needs, while private schools do not even have that sense of obligation.

The schools that traditionally do well on rankings such as that of *U.S. News* tended to be at the bottom of the social mission list. They are overwhelmingly private (14 of the bottom 20) and generally highly NIH-funded. Comments from the leaders of those schools, unsurprisingly, tended to disparage the study and its methods, and to assert, essentially, that "our school does well on all of its missions." This may well be so, provided that those missions do not include the social missions of meeting the health needs of the American people by producing minority and primary care physicians, and doctors who practice in underserved areas. In addition, these rankings are all relative, and while some are better than others, no medical schools (except the historically black schools and the Puerto Rican schools) are doing very well at producing minority physicians or physicians for rural areas at anything approaching the percent of Americans who live in those areas.

The data produced by the MEFS researchers showing that schools which are historically highly ranked do relatively poorly in social mission is not due to a flawed methodology. "The level of NIH support that medical schools received was inversely associated with their output of primary care physicians and physicians practicing in underserved areas." It is because at their best, these schools hardly integrate the characteristics that MEFS is measuring or the concept of social mission. Therefore, they do not put as much energy, time, or especially money into them. Mullan et al. write:

> *Some schools may choose other priorities, but in this time of national reconsideration, it seems appropriate that all schools examine their educational commitment regarding the service needs of their states and the nation. A diverse, equitably distributed physician workforce with a strong primary care base is essential to achieve quality health care that is accessible and affordable, regardless of the nature of any future health care reform.* [11]

Medical schools are the only institutions in our society that can produce physicians. It is up to the people of the U.S., particularly the communities in need and the policy makers who represent them, to decide how high a priority it is to produce physicians who will meet our social need. It is up to us to decide how to use the public coffers to achieve this. The time is long past, however, for these characteristics not to be measured. We can no longer, in self-indulgence or ignorance, assume that those schools that are the "best" on *U.S. News* rankings because of NIH research funding, selectivity, and "reputation" are the best in every area. The *U.S. News* rankings do not in any way account for social mission. In producing the doctors most needed by this nation's most needy, its most highly-ranked schools, are with few exceptions, the worst.

Community Based Medical Schools

Medical schools can have a positive impact on public health—if they set their minds to it. Because of the concern about lack of community responsiveness in traditional medical schools, there have been two rounds of creating "community-based" medical schools, the first in the late 1960s and early 1970s and the second in the 2000s. These schools differ from traditional academic health centers (AHCs) in that they do not have their own university hospital but rather use existing hospitals in the community to train students. In addition, they frequently have more of a community focus than traditional AHCs, usually have more concern for a social mission—meeting the common health needs of the community in which they are located—and are less focused on being the most sophisticated medical referral center or scientific research center in their region or nationally. That the first wave came out of the social action movements of the 1960s and 1970s is unsurprising. While many of the schools created then have maintained to a greater or lesser degree a focus on community health, many others have largely abandoned those missions as they have sought to replicate the Hopkins model and become major research centers. The creation of the newest group of community-based medical schools was in part a response to this situation, and a recognition that the need for doctors well-trained in the community continued to exist.

In 2012, community-based schools from both "generations" were featured at a Tulsa conference called *Beyond Flexner*, co-sponsored by the School of Community Medicine of the University of Oklahoma at Tulsa, the Medical Education Futures Study at George Washington University and the Josiah Macy Jr. Foundation. The successes achieved by the "first wave" of community-based schools were illustrated by presentations from the Morehouse School of Medicine, Southern Illinois University (SIU) School of Medicine, and the University of New Mexico (UNM) School of Medicine. Expectations for the future were presented by three schools of the "second wave", A.T. Still School of Osteopathic Medicine in Arizona, Northern Ontario School of Medicine, and the University of Oklahoma School of Community Medicine.

The three older schools are among those from that "first wave" that have done a better job of maintaining community focus, although they are quite different from each other. UNM (like a sizeable portion of the schools from that era) is not a community-based school, as it has its own large teaching hospital, and also has a very large research infrastructure and program. It does, however, also maintain a community focus; its *Vision 2020* statement is "The University of New Mexico Health Sciences Center will work with community partners to help New Mexico make more progress in health and health equity than any other state by 2020"; its mission statement echoes this, saying that "As a majority-minority state, our mission will ensure that all populations in New Mexico have access to the highest quality health care," and its first goal is to "Improve health and health care to the populations we serve with community-wide solutions."[12]

The newer medical schools have different backgrounds and

emphases. The Tulsa school is a branch of the traditional allopathic AHC of the University of Oklahoma in Oklahoma City, but specifically calls itself the "School of Community Medicine." A.T. Still in Arizona is an osteopathic school, and a new branch of the oldest school of osteopathic medicine in the U.S. It has an innovative curriculum that includes dispersing its students for clinical experiences to 20 Federally-Qualified Health Centers (FQHCs) across the country. Northern Ontario is, obviously, a Canadian school, the 6th medical school in that province, with two centers in Sudbury and Thunder Bay. It was created particularly to meet the rural health needs of its region.

If the *Beyond Flexner* conference actually becomes a movement, it will develop goals, standards and measurements for community accountability and a social mission. I suggest that these foci become core parts of it:

- *Diversity*: How does the school produce a health workforce that looks more like America by enrolling, and supporting, a group of students that is truly diverse in ethnicity, gender, socioeconomic status, and geographic origin?
- *Social Determinants of Health*: How does the school teach about and train students in, and carry out programs aimed at addressing, the social determinants of health? How does its curriculum and work invert that of the traditional medical school, which is focused most on tertiary hospital-care, to emphasize instead ambulatory care and community-based interventions to have an impact on the most important health determinants including housing, safety, education, food, and warmth?
- *Disparities*: How does the school, through its programs of ed-

ucation and community intervention, and its research agenda and practices, work to reduce disparities in health care and health among populations?

- *Community Engagement*: How does the school identify the community(ies) it serves and how does it involve them in determining the location of training, kinds of programs it carries out, and in identifying the questions that need to be answered by research?

The bottom line is that outcomes matter more than words, and that judging a school by the impact that it has on the health of the population should be the gold standard.

Who is Admitted to Medical School? Who Should Be?

Now we consider how medical schools perceive themselves, and how they do—or do not—produce primary care physicians. The experience that students have in medical school, both the formal curriculum and the "informal" (or "hidden") curriculum—that is, what people say, and the messages that students receive that are not included in the syllabus—have a major impact on student career choice, and it is one of the two large areas that the school and its faculty have control over. The other is the choice of students who are admitted to the school, because this may be an even more important determining factor in specialty choice.

If we compare the production of doctors to an industrial process, who is admitted is the "input variable", and the medical school experience is the "process variable." There is, of course, another critical factor, the "output variable": what is the experience of physicians in different specialties when they are in practice? What is their lifestyle like, how much money do they make, what is their social status? However, this last, while possibly the most important in affecting specialty choice, is not in the direct control of the schools in the way that the other variables are.

It would probably come as no surprise to most people that, on average, medical students generally come from privileged backgrounds. They come from upper-income families, with 80% from the top 20% of income. They come overwhelmingly from urban and suburban areas, and are disproportionately white and Asian (particularly South Asian), with a dramatic underrepresentation of African-Americans, Hispanics, Native Americans, Alaskan Natives, and Pacific Islanders. Also unsurprisingly, they have high grades, both in their college coursework and on the Medical College Admissions Test (MCAT) that all applicants take. It is this last characteristic that is sometimes presented as the justification for having medical school classes that look so different from the overall population; admissions committees and schools will say "we are just taking the best and the brightest." That rationale tends to resonate; after all, who wants a stupid doctor?

But, of course, there is a lot more to the issue than this. For starters, there is very close correlation between many of these characteristics. Students from well-to-do families, educated through high school at top private or suburban public schools, with wide-ranging opportunities and a plethora of advanced placement courses, will have better preparation for academics, get into more selective colleges and perform better on standardized tests. This is a key inequity, related to the same issues as the social determinants of health: those who come from privilege have great advantages and are likely to maintain those privileges; social mobility in the U.S. is very limited, as is increasingly being documented in both the popular press and in scientific economic literature.[13] More important, these characteristics that are most associated with admission to medical school are also associated with a significantly lower likelihood of entering primary care. The characteristics associated with a greater probability of entering primary care have been well-studied: rural background, member of an underrepresented minority group, older at the time of matriculation, and family of origin with lower socioeconomic status. And, because they are highly correlated, lower grades and MCAT scores.

Is this a true conundrum? Do we need to take "less qualified" students into medical school, do we need to "dumb down" our curriculum, to get more primary care doctors? No, not at all, because this approach takes a uni-dimensional view of "qualified", one which is not actually highly correlated with the important outcomes of medical education: how good are the doctors? What type of medicine do they practice and where do they practice it? Most important, how does this affect the health of the people?

These are the really important questions, and they take the issue of who should be admitted to medical school out of the realm of considering the individual who is "rewarded" for having high grades with the opportunity to become a doctor, to the realm of the society, which has a stake in who medical students are and what they will become. Is there a difference? Yes. For example, I might argue that a student who becomes a doctor who practices in a geographic area and in a specialty that already has sufficient (or even excess) supply, and cares for the segment of the population that already has sufficient (or even excess) access to medical care, is providing no marginal benefit to society. Why should we take a student with these goals into medical school? To turn the usual saw about taking students with lower grades on its head, is this not "wasting a seat"? That they may be able to make a very good income in what seems an adequately-supplied market is a testimony to the nature of medical practice, where to a large extent supply drives demand rather than the converse.

Ultimately even a suburban, upscale market may become super-saturated and no longer be fertile ground for new specialists, but while waiting for this to correct there remain huge populations with little or no access at all. On the other hand, the student who wants to practice primary care in an underserved area (either rural or urban), and whose practice plans are about improving access for those who have too little, is much more likely to make a difference in the health of the public, and thus should be considered more qualified for medical school. Yes, academic performance is important, but it cannot and should not be the sole criterion. It will lead to—what it has led to—a society with large portions of the population without sufficient access to care, a specialty to primary care ratio turned on its head. Every system is perfectly designed to get the results that it gets.

Does this mean that we don't want the smartest people we can to become doctors? No, but it does require that the definition of smart and capable include characteristics that extend beyond grades. When we look simply at prior academic performance, those with better preparation will usually perform better in the pre-clinical years, but it doesn't mean that they are necessarily smarter or more capable. There are students who get into medical school and initially struggle because their prior preparation has been less rigorous, but who with time and experience outperform some of those students who have had all the advantages—educated parents, excellent high schools, tutoring when needed.

More to the point, there are few or no data, either from studies or anecdotally, that correlate higher academic performance in the pre-medical setting with quality of performance in the clinical arena, whether in medical school or in later practice. There is some correlation with higher grades in the pre-clinical, basic science curriculum, which is not surprising since those courses mirror the same kind of courses that the students did well in previously. However, when working with patients enters into the equation, this correlation no longer holds. Here we have a need to be able to interact effectively with people, to communicate with them, to be able to translate medical information into something that they can understand and use to make decisions about their health. Students need to be able to listen, to really hear what people's concerns are, to know how to address them, and to be able to reach a solution that meets the needs of the patient, and not just insist on what the physician knows to be "right." This is an entirely separate set of skills, and without them, most physicians, at least those who are in specialties that directly interact with living, awake patients, will be less than competent.

Even in the "academic" realm, the skills that are required to do well in pre-med and the classroom years of medical school are largely dependent on success in remembering facts and being able to repeat them back when being tested. But this is less important than in past years because the increase in medical knowledge and the rate at which it changes are beyond the capacity of any person to keep up with, and because technology has made this information available on demand. What is needed for an effective physician is the ability to integrate information into a usable plan, to solve problems, and to make decisions in settings where the information is incomplete or the benefits ambiguous. The preferences—and resources—of the patient also have to be taken into account. This is highly difficult, very challenging, absolutely necessary, and not particularly related to the ability to regurgitate facts.

Ensuring that we have an equitable society in which people of all social, ethnic, and economic backgrounds have equality of opportunity for at least a fine education, and thus the preparation for excellent performance, is a long-term challenge that needs to be taken seriously. In the meantime, however, we need to be sure that we do not multiply the discrimination in selection of medical students by not considering all characteristics of applicants, including problem solving skills, communication skills, empathy, goals for their practice (in terms of what populations they hope to care for) and a commitment to social justice as well as grades. The entire concept of "qualified" in regard to higher education in general is addressed in an excellent book by law professors Lani Guinier and Susan Sturm, aptly titled *Who's Qualified?* They argue, as I do, that the issue is not one of taking less-qualified students, but rather reconsidering what "qualified" means, and looking at it from a societal rather than individual perspective.[14]

This discussion has so far not addressed the issue of "diversity" in medical school students as a value in itself, but rather has stressed that the criteria by which students are currently selected for medical school do not reflect the skills that are needed to become effective physicians. Expanding these criteria to look at the overall skills and experience of applicants, and recognizing that higher grades do not predict being a better doctor so that these receive lower emphasis in the admissions process, is likely to broaden the economic, ethnic, and geographic makeup of these classes, and to lead to a population of students who are more likely to meet the needs of the American people by their practice. Underserved people are more likely to be from poorer, minority and rural backgrounds and settings, so that training doctors from those backgrounds is more likely to result in people who choose to care for them. This is not only common sense, but has been shown by the results of small programs which have recruited students from rural backgrounds who are in fact much more likely to practice in rural areas[15,16] and by studies showing that minority physicians are much more likely to practice with ethnic minority populations.[17,18]

Diversity in medical school classrooms is in itself of value. It is of value for students to recognize that other people have had different life experiences, have had to overcome different barriers, and may not been have been able to rely on the same presumption of a safety net that they have. Sharing experiences in medical school, in small groups and maybe even in voluntary study groups, broadens understanding and increases the capability to work with patients whose background is different from one's own. It helps to see both what is possible and what the obstacles might be, and makes for a better doctor.

There are, of course, many upper-income, white, suburban students who can and will become excellent doctors by whatever measure, including choosing primary care specialties and providing care to underserved populations. The challenge, however, is in assessing their applications prior to selection. An essay indicating intention is obviously too easy to fake if the applicant knows that this is what is being valued. Selection criteria need to include past behaviors, which are the best predictors of future behaviors. Were applicants in the Peace Corps, or VISTA, or Teach for America? Did they carry the rape crisis pager in college? Were they involved in setting up or staffing a free clinic? Did their volunteer work demonstrate a protracted commitment? What, in essence, is their social mission resume? Absent these characteristics, then students without the demographic predictors above should be considered with caution. By the same token, there will be many students who are from low income, minority, rural backgrounds who will become subspecialists and practice in affluent communities. That the demographic characteristic increases the likelihood of primary care and underserved practice does not guarantee it, nor should it. These students should have the same opportunity to choose specialties as others.

Thus, on the front end, there needs to be major change in our "input variable" in who is accepted into medical school.

The Content of the Medical School Curriculum: The Gap Between What is Taught and What Students Need to Know

Beyond the "input variable" for medical education—the students who are selected—the other big area that medical educators have control over is the "process variable"—the medical school curriculum. The curriculum in most medical schools is divided into two parts; the first two years (more or less) are devoted to "basic science" education in anatomy, physiology, biochemistry, pharmacology, and microbiology. This is largely classroom (lecture and, increasingly, small-group) and laboratory learning, not very different from the experience students have had previously in college. It is punctuated by a national examination, the U.S. Medical Licensing Examination (USMLE) Step 1, which focuses on these "basic sciences." The last two years (more or less) are spent in clinical training, often in the hospital, with both required experiences in a number of specialties (commonly internal medicine, surgery, family medicine, pediatrics, psychiatry, obstetrics-gynecology, and neurology) along with other required and elective experiences.

Over the decades, there have been modifications to this. Increasingly, encouraged by the Liaison Committee for Medical Education (LCME, which accredits medical schools), clinical experiences are being included in the first two years, together with a greater proportion of small group learning and teaching of some material that is less "biologic science" and more "social science" including ethics, determinants of health, and epidemiology. Many schools have decreased the number of months in the basic science years, so that clinical experiences start earlier. However, while these changes have taken place, often with resistance from some of the faculty, the core Flexnerian principle of basic science followed by clinical training remains the norm.

There is, however, good reason to question this long-standing model. The faculty members who teach and define the first part of the medical school curriculum are largely non-physician scientists who are primarily researchers. They are often working at the cutting edge of scientific discovery, creating new knowledge, while the knowledge that medical students need in their education is much more basic, much more about understanding the scientific method and what constitutes valid evidence. There is relatively little need, at this stage, for students to learn about the current research that these scientists are doing. This curriculum has been heavily laden with memorization of lots of facts, details about basic cell structure and function and other areas. The burden and challenge of fact memorization has become the meme by which people characterize medical school. It is also probably unnecessary. After 5 years of non-use students likely retain only 10% of what they learn; even if they need 10%—or more—in their future careers, there is no likelihood that the 10% they retain will be the 10% they need.[19]

Of course, these scientists not only teach medical students, they (or their colleagues at other institutions) write the questions for USMLE Step 1. This creates a tautology: basic science faculty can persuasively argue that students need to learn what they teach because it is on the exam, and the exam is created by them to assess this knowledge. The criterion of "do all doctors need to know this, and will learning it at this stage of their careers improve health care?" isn't a concern.

In order for our society to have a more appropriate set of doctors, medical schools and the LCME have to do a better job of determining what portion of the information currently taught in the "basic sciences" is crucial for all future doctors to know and memorize. We also need to broaden the definition of "basic science" to include the key social sciences of anthropology, sociology, psychology, communication, and even many areas of the humanities, such as ethics. This is not likely to happen in a curriculum controlled by molecular biologists. There are a number of areas not part of the biological sciences that students need to learn, or if they already know it, have fostered rather than extinguished (whether intentionally or not) while they are in medical school. Two of these are *communication* and *empathy*.

Training Doctors to be Great Communicators and to Have Empathy

When asked, most medical students start school with some desire to help people, and sometimes even to help humanity. They often change later, and they frequently have little concrete idea of what this would mean. They are generally from more affluent, urban backgrounds, but a large percentage of them do want to make a difference. They speak English as other people in the United States and are able to communicate effectively. However, there has long been a sense that the medical school experience, rather than building on and nurturing these values, has the opposite effect. For students who enter with less commitment, the negative impact is even greater. A 2009 study demonstrated an appalling drop in empathy among medical students as they go through school. Empathy stays relatively constant from matriculation to the end of their second year, but drops to reach a nadir in their third (first clinical) year. There is something of a rebound in their fourth year, but nowhere near enough to bring them back to where they were when they started.[20] This is disturbing, but the real question is: Why? Only if we can answer this can we try to address it.

In the study that demonstrated attrition of empathy, students were given the opportunity to identify themselves so that data could be analyzed over time for individuals or groups of individuals as well as the whole group. Unfortunately, only 25% did, so looking at trends among sub-groups, which could only be done on this smaller group, provides less robust data. However, within this "matched" group, women started with higher empathy scores than did men and dropped less, although still significantly. In addition, students who planned to enter "technology-oriented" specialties (anesthesiology, pathology, radiology, surgery, orthopedics, etc.) not only had greater drops in their empathy scores than those entering "people-oriented" specialties (family medicine, internal medicine, pediatrics, emergency medicine, psychiatry, obstetrics and gynecology), but had lower scores to begin with. This means that, at least among this group who allowed themselves to be tracked, there is a difference in empathy levels even at baseline, at entry, between those entering the different types of specialties (when taken as a group). A comparable study was done in Japan, and Japanese students did not demonstrate this decline; the reasons are presumably cultural.[21]

The difference in empathy scores between entering medical students (the "input variable") based on the specialty they finally choose is interesting, if not surprising, and suggests that greater attention to these characteristics could increase the number of students entering primary care. The attrition of empathy in all students through medical school, however, is a process variable. It has been suggested that the constant interaction with people with severe health problems "hardens" students, and that seeing people who students perceive have brought those problems on themselves by their behaviors can decrease their empathy. Clearly, if this is not desirable, there must be conscious attention paid to it in the medical school curriculum.

Effective communication provides a similar challenge—students presumably enter with the ability to talk to other people so that they can be understood, but their ability to do so decreases as they go through medical school. As they struggle to acculturate to the profession, part of what they need to learn is a new language that is replete with eponyms, abbreviations, and long abstruse names for diseases (many are from Latin, and while they are impressive and complicated, they are also sometimes trite in translation, e.g., "erythema" means "red", "pruritic" means "itchy"). They have to learn to speak "medical" so that they can understand and talk with their supervisors, both residents and attending physicians, as a way to be accepted into the guild by their seniors. But as they learn this new language, they must be careful that it does not block their ability to communicate with their patients. They also need to continue to speak English (or whatever the language is that their patients speak) in the vernacular, so that they can effectively communicate.

Something that is experienced by many new doctors, and even medical students, is that (provided they do not come from a medical family) they become presumptive medical experts for their family and friends. It happened to me and I have discussed it with generations of students, and most laugh with embarrassment as they acknowledge receiving such calls from virtually the moment they received their acceptance letters. Telling people that they don't know anything yet doesn't stop the calls, because the people who are calling are often looking for something different from real medical knowledge. Rather than medical advice, they are looking for a translation of what their doctor has told them, and think that someone they know can help them to understand. "I may have particularly stupid family and friends, or their doctors may be particularly bad," I tell the students, "but I don't think so. The first part of most of my conversations is trying to discover what their doctor might have told them that led them to *think* that what they are telling me is what their doctor told them. While it might not always be true, if you assume that *no one* understood *anything* their doctor told them, you'd be right more often than wrong."

It is unfortunate if this is the situation for communication between doctors and patients, but it is often the case. Words that physicians would never even think of as being related, except in a part of their etymology that no one in the profession pays attention to, sound similar to regular people and can lead to confusion. "Orthopedic" or "orthodontic"? One is about bones and one about teeth, but to a non-medical person they sound a great deal alike. In addition, physicians and nurses use a lot of non-specific and unfamiliar words like "lesion" and "vital signs" and "lab values" and "blood tests" and "foreign body." Goodness! Is it any wonder that studies have shown lots of people have no idea what it means to have a "foreign body in your eye"? "Something in your eye" is not only comprehensible, it is no less meaningful. Indeed, sometimes "medical" meanings seem to be the opposite of normal speech; we talk of "negative" results as good (nothing bad was found) and "positive" results as bad (we found something bad). Is it any wonder that people are confused?

Sometimes the vagueness of speaking "medical" may be part of a different problem, making the doctor or student more comfortable providing bad news, because it offers a convenient way to obscure and temporize. If we say that "the biopsy indicates a malignant neoplasm" instead of "you have cancer" we may not consciously be trying to avoid a difficult conversation, but that can be the result. Of course, it confuses the patient. We may rationalize this by saying "what I said is more technically true; we're not 100% sure it is cancer", or "I am trying to be gentle and not cruel to the patient." But for the patient this line of discussion can be completely meaningless.

There is a skill in being able to care for other people, while retaining empathy for them, even when they frequently don't do what you advise them to do, and even when you don't understand their life circumstances and how they affect them, and how you would react in a similar setting. There is a skill in knowing medicine, of being able to speak medical and being able to converse in this language with your peers and seniors, while retaining the ability to translate that information and those concepts into language that people who are not medical can understand and use. These are skills that can be learned, and need to be developed and nurtured. These skills, far more than memorization of enzyme pathways or cell structure, are what help physicians to help patients.

The Contribution of Medical School Culture
to the Primary Care Crisis

Researchers at the Association of American Medical Colleges (AAMC) have looked at aspects of medical school culture that influence student specialty choice. They surveyed all 4th-year medical students from a random sample of 20 medical schools to assess both student and school level characteristics that were associated with greater likelihood of entering primary care. The most important finding was that only 13% of these final-year medical students were planning on primary care careers, even though 40% were planning to enter the ostensibly "primary care" residencies of internal medicine (IM), pediatrics (PD), family medicine (FM), and internal medicine-pediatrics (IM/PD).[22]

What explains the difference? Most of it results from students entering internal medicine residencies (which "count" as primary care) with the intention of going on to subspecialization (e.g., in cardiology or gastroenterology or endocrinology) and thus having no intention of actually practicing primary care. While this provides further evidence that the medical school practice (supported historically by AAMC) of reporting "primary care" rates by entry into residencies in those fields is not valid, the much more important finding is the degree to which it demonstrates the extent of the problem. A 13% production rate of primary care physicians will not get us up to the 30% to 40% (or 50%) primary care that is needed no matter how long we wait; obviously it will take us in the other direction.

The main outcome variable of the AAMC study was entry into primary care, and it specifically looked at two school-level (as perceived by the students in the survey) characteristics: "bad-mouthing" primary care (faculty, residents or other students saying, for example, that primary care is a fall-back or something that is a "waste of a mind") and having a greater than the average number of positive primary care experiences. It turns out that both were associated with primary care choice, in opposite directions. Having a larger number of positive primary care experiences was associated with greater choice of a primary care career. In the case of badmouthing, students from schools with higher than average reported rates were less likely to be planning primary care careers. However, those students from the schools with a higher rate of badmouthing who *were* planning primary care careers reported higher rates of badmouthing than those who were not; perhaps this is because they were more sensitive to it. Altogether, though, after controlling for individual student and school characteristics, these factors accounted for only 8% of the difference in primary care choice. Consistent with the discussion above on the importance of who is admitted to medical school, characteristics of the student (demographics such as sex, minority status or rural origin, academic performance defined as the score on Step 1 of USMLE, as well as expectation of income and feeling of a personal "fit" with primary care), and of the school (research emphasis, private vs. public, selectivity) accounted for the rest. Interestingly, debt was not a significant factor in this study.[23]

As discussed above, many of these individual and school characteristics are highly correlated. A school that prides itself on being selective (taking students with high scores) and producing subspecialists and research scientists does not have to badmouth primary care—the institutional culture implicitly marginalizes it. On the other side, the students selected at those schools are more likely to have those characteristics (particularly high socioeconomic status and urban or suburban origin) not associated with students who make the primary care choice. It is worth noting that the measure of academic performance in this study was USMLE Step 1, usually taken after the first 2 years and focusing more on the basic science material covered in those years, rather than USMLE Step 2, which covers more clinical material. This biases the assessment of academic qualification. Both pre-medical grades and scores on the Medical College Admissions Test (MCAT) are highly correlated with pre-clinical medical school course grades and USMLE Step 1 scores, but they are not correlated with performance in any clinical activity.

Therefore, a large part of the problem of too few students entering primary care specialties is in the overall culture of medical schools, their perception of what their role should be (creating research scientists vs. clinicians, creating subspecialists vs. primary care doctors), and in their belief that taking students with the highest grades is equivalent to taking the best students. If the goal is indeed to increase the number of primary care doctors, this culture, because it has undesirable outcomes for the production of the doctors America needs, must change.

If we trained doctors in the right way in the right place we might have a better shot at getting the health system, and even the health, our country needs.

References

1   Mullan F, Chen C, Petterson S, Kolsky G et al. The social mission of medical educa-
    tion: ranking the schools, *Ann Intern Med* 152(12):804-811, 2010.

2   Flexner, A. *Medical Education in the United States and Canada.* Carnegie Founda-
    tion for the Advancement of Teaching. Bulletin #4. New York. 1910.

3   White, K L Williams, TF, Greenberg, BC. The ecology of medical care. *N Engl J Med
    265: 885-892, 1961.*

4   Green, LA et al. The ecology of medical care revisited, *N Engl J Med 344: 2021-
    2025, 2001.*

5   Ibid # 4.

6   *Gladwell, M. David and Goliath: Underdogs, Misfits, and the Art of Battling Giants.*
    Little, Brown. New York. 2013.

7   Flanigan, S., Morse, R., Medical School Rankings Methodology - How we rank
    medical schools. *U.S. News and World Report*, April, 22, 2009. http://www.us-
    news.com/education/articles/2009/04/22/medical-school-rankings-methodology

8   Garibaldi, RA, Popkave C, Bylsma W, Career plans for trainees in internal medicine
    residency programs, *Acad Med* 80(5):507-12, May, 2005

9   Hauer KE, Durning SJ, Kernan WN et al., Factors associated with medical students'
    career choices regarding internal medicine. *JAMA* 300(10):1154-64, 2008

10 Medical Education Futures Study, Beyond Flexner: the social mission of medicine.
    http://www.medicaleducationfutures.org/projects/beyond-flexner

11 Ibid #1.

12 University of New Mexico Health Science Center. Vision, Mission, and Core Values.
    http://hsc.unm.edu/about/mission.shtml

13 Piketty, T. *Capital in the Twenty-First Century* (English translation). *Belknap Press.*
    Cambridge, MA. 2014.

14 Guinier L and Sturm S. *Who's Qualified?. Beacon Press.* Boston. 2001.

15 Rabinowitz HK, Diamond JJ, Markham FW et al. Retention of rural family physi-
    cians after 20-25 years: outcomes of a comprehensive medical school rural pro-
    gram. *J Am Board Fam Med* 26(1):24-7, Jan-Feb, 2013.

16 Zink T, Center B, Finstad D et al. Efforts to graduate more primary care physicians
    and physicians who will practice in rural areas: examining outcomes from the Uni-

versity of Minnesota-Duluth and the rural physician associate program. *Acad Med* 85(4):599-604, April 12, 2010

17   Walker KO, Moreno G, Grumbach K. The association among specialty, race, ethnicity, and practice location among California physicians in diverse specialties. *J Natl Med Assoc.* 104(1-2):46-52, Jan-Feb, 2012.

18   Grumbach K, Hart LG, Mertz E et al. Who is caring for the underserved? A comparison of primary care physicians and non-physician clinicians in California and Washington. *Ann Fam Med* 1(2):97-104. Jul-Aug, 2003

19   McGaghie W, Miller GE, Sajid AW et al. Competency-based curriculum development in medical education: an introduction. *Public Health Papers* #68. World Health Organization. Geneva. 1978.

20   Hojat M, Vergare MJ, Maxwell K, et al, The Devil is in the Third Year: A Longitudinal Study of Erosion of Empathy in Medical School, *Academic Medicine*, 84(2):1182-91, Sept, 2009

21   Kataoka HU, Koide N, Ochi K et al. Measurement of empathy among Japanese medical students: psychometrics and score differences by gender and level of medical education, *Academic Medicine* 84(9):1192-7, Sept. 2009.

22   Erikson CE, Danish S, Jones KC et al. The role of in medical school culture in primary care career choice, *Acad Med.* 88(12):1919-26. Dec., 2013.

23   Ibid # 22.

Chapter 7

After Medical School:
Residency Training

Primary care physician production of 25.2% and rural physician production of 4.8% will not sustain the current workforce, solve problems of maldistribution, or address acknowledged shortages.[1]

—Candice Chen, M.D. and colleagues

The process of educating and training physicians has two distinct phases: medical school, at the end of which students receive an M.D. (or D.O., in schools of osteopathic medicine), which can be thought of as the production of undifferentiated physicians. Following medical school graduation, new doctors then train for several years in their specialty (depending upon the specialty and any subspecialty, 3 to 7 or more years) to become internists, psychiatrists, pediatricians, family doctors, obstetrician/gynecologists, general surgeons, anesthesiologists, neurologists, radiologists, pathologists, orthopedists, urologists, plastic surgeons, otolaryngologists, ophthalmologists, emergency physicians, etc., and any of the subspecialties of these areas. The most familiar subspecialties in internal medicine, such as cardiology, endocrinology, gastroenterology, etc., take two or more additional years beyond the three for internal medicine. The primary care specialties are family medicine (FM), general internal medicine (GIM), and general pediatrics (GP), which as a rule are 3 year residencies, and a combined internal medicine-pediatrics residency (IM/PD) which is usually 4 years. Family medicine programs are the most similar to each other. While a graduate of any internal medicine program can practice as a generalist, there are some internal medicine programs that are particularly targeted at primary care, with greater emphasis on ambulatory care and continuity of care than the more typical hospital-focused internal medicine program.

In Chapter 5 on Primary Care, I discussed the benefits to societies of an adequate representation of primary care doctors (and other primary care providers such as primary care nurse practitioners and physician's assistants) as a proportion of all physicians and other providers who practice in other specialty areas. I also noted that the U.S., in contrast to most other industrialized countries, has a skewed ratio, with fewer than 30% primary care providers, and that the trend is downwards, particularly in internal medicine. In the last chapter, I addressed a number of complex issues that have an impact on this process, which include what I call "input variables" (who do we take in medical school?), "process variables" (what is their experience, including the formal and informal curriculum, while in school?), and "output variables" (what is the practice environment, including workload, personal satisfaction, status and of course income?) I noted that the first two are much more controllable by medical schools, but the last is really an issue for the entire health system, and indeed the broader society. In addition, there are policy issues, in particular the funding for residency training (Graduate Medical Education, or GME). Most of the cost of this training is paid for by Medicare ($9.5 billion in 2011)[2] and Medicaid ($3.2 billion in 2012)[3], and how it might be expanded, modified, or cut has a major impact on residency training.

What about the future? Is there any evidence to help us estimate the likely future mix of specialists? A recent study by Chen
and colleagues looked at how institutions that sponsor GME (and
get those large amounts of money from Medicare and Medicaid)
do in producing specialists in short supply.[4] The authors define
these as primary care physicians (family medicine [FM], general
internal medicine [GIM], general pediatrics [GP], combined internal medicine–pediatrics [IM/PD], internal medicine geriatrics
[IM-G], and family medicine geriatrics [FM-G]), general surgeons, obstetrician-gynecologists, and psychiatrists. Identifying
which institution produced whom is quite a bit harder than when
looking at medical school outcomes. GME-sponsoring institutions can be a hospital, consortium of a medical school and one
or more hospitals, or even a non-profit organization set up for that
purpose. They may often sponsor more than one residency program in the same specialty.

As in all studies that look at primary care production, the big
variable is in internal medicine programs, the majority of whose
graduates go into subspecialty (e.g., cardiology, gastroenterology,
pulmonary and critical care) fellowships rather than remaining in
primary care/general internal medicine (GIM). This study takes
pains to account for this variable, and notes that their figure of an
average of 25.2% of internal medicine graduates entering primary
care "…overestimates primary care production, as we could not
account for primary care physicians practicing as hospitalists."
Hospitalists are physicians, usually in internal medicine or pediatrics or family medicine, whose practice consists entirely of caring
for hospitalized patients; they do not practice in the ambulatory
setting and are clearly not in primary care. By many accounts they
may represent a majority of those completing the basic internal

medicine training but not going on to fellowship.

Just as there is a wide variation in the percent of medical school graduates entering primary care residency programs, this study found a wide variation in the percent of graduates of different sponsoring institutions who entered these specialties-in-need. Of 759 sponsoring institutions, they "...found that 158 institutions produced no primary care graduates, and 184 institutions produced more than 80%; the latter tended to be smaller institutions." Again no surprise; the larger, often more famous and "elite" sponsoring institutions (most often hospitals associated with elite medical schools) did a terrible job at producing the physicians the nation needs most. Smaller sponsoring institutions—often hospitals with one (usually family medicine) or a few residencies, in smaller cities and towns, and affiliated with Federally-Qualified Health Centers (FQHCs) or Area Health Education Centers (AHECs), based in in underserved urban and rural communities, did well. The Robert Graham Center website (www.graham-center.org) provides interactive tools to allow you to map the density of primary care physicians by state, county and other areas, the output of each institution producing residents in terms of location and specialty, and the footprint of graduates from each GME program.

It is worth restating that 158 institutions sponsoring graduate medical education produced *no* primary care graduates. Some other numbers from the study:

- 198 institutions (more than 25% of the total) produced *no* rural physicians, while only 10 institutions had all graduates go to rural areas;
- the average percentage of graduates providing direct patient care in rural areas was 4.8% (the rural population of the U.S., for comparison, is about 20%).

- 283 institutions (37%) produced *no* physicians practicing in FQHCs or rural health clinics (RHCs); 479 (63%) of institutions produced no physicians for the National Health Service Corps (NHSC), a program for sponsoring physicians for underserved areas).[5]

These outcomes can be explained by Batalden's Law that every system is perfectly designed to get the results that it gets. Our graduate medical education system is designed so that hospitals sponsoring GME programs will have the (cheap) resident staff in areas that generate higher income for the institution, that ensure the adequate production of future high-profit-margin specialists for the institution, and that attract high income (or at least well-insured) patients. It is not designed to ensure that all Americans have access to the doctors that they need.

Elite academic medical centers have values that lead them to attract and select students and trainees with characteristics that are the opposite of those needed for training physicians to meet the needs of the American people. They value caring for rarer and highly specialized conditions, which are both highly reimbursed and provide the basis for research in narrow areas of disease (and almost never of health). They value receiving large sums of money from the National Institutes of Health (NIH) for research, most of which is basic laboratory research. These are not bad things; they are, in fact, necessary. We need research, including basic laboratory research and first-in-human studies, for medical science to advance, although we also need a lot more funding for population-based research into the causes of health and disease, and community-based efforts to address them. We need tertiary-care medical centers where rare or more complex conditions can be most effectively treated by physicians and surgeons whose narrower expertise makes them more experienced and effective.

The problem is that concentrating all these subspecialists in the very places where students and residents are trained gives those learners a very skewed idea of the ratio of subspecialists to primary care doctors, and makes the teachers want to attract the "best" students to go into their narrow, subspecialized areas. In addition, selection for medical school (and to a large extent for residencies that are more competitive because they have fewer slots) tend to be for students who have the characteristics that help them to do well in basic science courses, standardized tests, and possibly in laboratory research. As described earlier, these students tend to come from high income families of professionals, in the largest metropolitan areas, from elite public or suburban schools. They look a great deal like the people who have plenty of doctors to care for them, and very little like the people whose communities suffer from a dearth of physicians, particularly in inner city and rural areas. That is, they look very little like the people who need the most care, not the wealthy but the poor. I have previously noted that, while about 20% of Americans live in rural areas, only about 9% of doctors practice in such areas, but Chen and colleagues's study shows it is actually getting much worse, with only 4.8% of graduates entering rural practice in 2012.[6]

The absence of a national workforce policy provides students the opportunity to choose a specialty based on what they believe, at the time they are making the decision, with the information that they have—will be best for them personally. Indeed, national health workforce policy in the U.S. is not defined by any analysis of future health needs with government programs providing incentives for students to enter the area of greatest need; rather it is defined by the perceived short-term self-interest of a group of relatively privileged young people. This situation is exacerbated by the inequity in income between primary care doctors and sub-specialists, an inequity also seen (albeit at a higher level) for general surgeons vs. subspecialty surgeons, especially when hours of work are considered. Thus students, generally selected from a population not representative of the American people, who have increasing debt (even for those from upper-middle-income, not to mention middle-income and the rare student from low income families), are attracted to specialties that pay the most. Many will even eschew specialties that pay well but require a lot of work (such as general surgery and orthopedic surgery) for those that pay the most for the least work (where income/work ratios are the highest). As predicted by Batalden's Law, this is a formula to continue what we have, not to make things better.

In recent years there has been a very significant expansion of U.S. medical schools. For the first time since the early 1970s, this century has seen an increase in the numbers of both allopathic and osteopathic schools. Existing schools are expanding their class size. The AAMC points out, correctly, that expanding medical school class size will not translate into more doctors if there are not more residency positions; it will likely decrease the number of international medical graduates obtaining those positions, but not create more doctors. AAMC is therefore calling for increasing the number of residency positions. This could be a great opportunity to increase the primary care workforce by calling for a requirement that a certain (large) percentage of those increases be in primary care. But the AAMC is not doing this. Their position may not be intended to be antagonistic toward primary care, but rather to show respect for all specialties that are represented by the AAMC.

Whatever the intention, such policies will at best create "more of the same" and not increase primary care. Indeed, the likely effect will be to worsen the problem. Since primary care residents are not big money-makers for the hospitals that are the main sponsors of residency training and primary care residency slots are not in great demand by medical students, it is quite likely that without specific requirements favoring primary care the opposite will occur—most of the expanded number of residency slots will be in non- primary care specialties. This will, of course, further exacerbate the already unbalanced subspecialty/primary care ratio.

Unlike the AAMC, many family medicine organizations are calling for expansion of residency slots to be tied to primary care, and I am in agreement with that. However, the concept of "forcing" students who may not want primary care residency slots into them makes many people uncomfortable. They would prefer to "make family medicine more desirable" to our students. This would be great, but would require major changes in reimbursement, a solution discussed later in this book. Indeed, there are many students who would choose family medicine as a specialty because of their interest in the work, but, with their debt load, find it hard to ignore a 2-3 times greater income in many other specialties

In addition to the income issues, students get the double message from many of their teachers both that primary care is "too hard" (because you have to know about everything) and that primary care is "too easy," (because you will not know "everything" about a particular area). If this seems contradictory, it is, but it is the reality in medical schools, an ironic conundrum. To the extent that student perceptions of specialties play a role in specialty choice, it can create a self-perpetuating cycle in which the specialties that are more competitive are perceived as not only of higher status, but "more difficult" and requiring greater skills.

Students choose to apply to residency programs in a particular specialty for a variety of reasons, including status, income potential, and what is often called lifestyle—as well as, one hopes, an interest in the work that those specialists do. When more students choose to apply to certain specialties than there are residency positions available, getting a position becomes more competitive. If, as is usually the case, the criteria for choosing residents in competitive programs is academic performance (grades and USMLE scores), then those specialties will have very high academic achievers, which can create a perception that, because you have to be "smart" (or at least have high grades) to get into a specialty, you have to be particularly smart to perform that specialty.

An example: recently a student who had wanted to enter a more "selective" specialty also applied (as is common) to family medicine as a "backup." S/he did not succeed in matching in her/his chosen first choice, but also did not match in family medicine. I don't know why, of course; perhaps it was because it was clear from her/his interviews that he s/he saw family medicine as a backup. However, the story that this person created (presumably to feel better) and shared with friends was that s/he was "too strong for family medicine." This may be an obvious self-justification, but in fact the story was brought to me by a friend who believed it to be true. More generally, it illustrates a flawed concept that conflates the difficulty of entry into a specialty with the complexity of the work done by specialists in that field. This can be true, but can also not be; it is difficult for a person from a war-torn region to gain entry to the U.S. as a refugee, but this doesn't make life harder in the U.S. than where they were. In this sense it is similar to the common self-justification used by people in privileged settings from high social caste to corporate boardrooms; rather than "I am here so I deserve to be here", it says "it was hard for me to get here, so it must be hard to do what I do."

I don't think it is possible for someone to be "too strong" for family medicine regardless of how you define strength (grades, board scores, compassion, ability to learn and apply learning, multi-tasking, or how much you can bench press). Indeed, I believe that family medicine is truly the most complex and difficult specialty. The breadth is enormous, as I am reminded each time I have to re-certify and must study maternity care, sports medicine, caring for people with heart disease, well-child care, ICU care, lung disease, diabetes, fractures, arthritis, acutely-ill children, preventive care, epidemiology, nutrition, gynecologic problems, management of psychiatric problems, adolescent issues, and on and on. There is nothing like it. It is also true that the skills, preferences, and experiences that make someone strong for one specialty may not make them "stronger" for another.

As far as the practice is concerned, family physicians see undifferentiated patients and try to come to a conclusion about what problems they have and how to manage them. This is a lot more conceptually challenging than seeing someone with a ready diagnosis or a narrow scope of diagnoses and applying your in-depth knowledge to figuring out a best method of treatment for it, or doing a procedure on it. Family physicians (and other primary care/generalist physicians) do not care for one disease or organ system of a person, they care for the person. They manage multiple co-existing chronic diseases. Our adult patients typically have a number of conditions such as hypertension, diabetes, heart disease, arthritis, depression, and social stressors in their lives.

The challenge is to balance the treatments for each so that they do not make the others worse and are best designed for that individual person. And, while doing so, to learn about and care for the person. This is harder than doing the same limited set of procedures or treating the same limited set of diagnoses day after day. Data derived from the National Ambulatory Medical Care Survey (NAMCS) of 2011 show that it takes 23 diagnoses to account for half of all the diagnoses a family physician cares for, while it takes only 8 for obstetrician-gynecologists, 6 for cardiologists, and 3 for psychiatrists.[7] This introduces great complexity, since a given person may have several diagnoses, and treating them is more complex than treating each one, involving both treating the ways both the diseases and the treatments for them might interact (e.g., will a drug to treat one disease make another one worse?).

I do not mean in any way to insult or seem to be critical of other specialists. They do important things and we need them to refer to as consultants for the procedures that we don't do, as well as the uncommon cases of diseases that are rarer or unresponsive to usual treatment. It is true that many other non-primary care specialties specialties require strong medical students. But it is incorrect to confuse supply/demand issues with the intelligence, hard work, difficulty, decision making ability needed, breadth, and conceptual complexity of a specialty. For these, nothing exceeds family medicine. If family medicine is difficult and complex, it is also rewarding for people who truly value the ability to have a relationship with a patient over time, and be responsible for their total health care. However, if the pay is not commensurate, it will continue to be difficult to attract a sufficient number of students into the discipline.

Chen and the other authors of the paper on GME accountability say that:

Primary care physician production of 25.2% and rural physician production of 4.8% will not sustain the current workforce, solve problems of maldistribution, or address acknowledged shortages. The relatively small number of physicians choosing to work in RHCs, FQHCs, HPSAs, and the NHSC will not support a doubling of the capacity of safety net services envisioned by the Affordable Care Act.[8]

They have that right. Medical schools and GME-sponsoring institutions have for too long been allowed to continue being self-serving, with the biggest institutions entirely pitiful in terms of producing the doctors America needs. Our graduate medical education system needs an immediate, far-reaching, large-scale change, where the biggest training programs see themselves in the business of producing primary care doctors for underserved people. What might encourage them to do that? For starters, the $9.5 billion in Medicare and $3.18 billion in Medicaid GME funding could be re-allocated to require outcomes that would benefit society rather than simply hospitals and AHCs.

There are some core functions and characteristics of primary care doctors that are very important to people. The doctors need to keep them in mind, their employers need to keep them in mind, insurers and policy makers need to keep them in mind. When health care is segmented into boxes that seem "rational" from a cost-allocation point of view (ambulatory doctors for this, hospitalists for that, emergency doctors for the other thing), we can lose the benefit of having a doctor who cares for us as a whole person. In the online medical literary journal *Pulse,* Steven Lewis writes of having a very scary health episode that takes him to the emergency room. He acutely feels the depersonalization of not having a doctor who knew him, like his old, now retired, doctor, Herb Weinman, did:

I know that the overworked ER staff who treated me were good and competent healthcare providers. But I also know that there was not a soul in the ER that day who would have cried if I had died. As Herb Weinman would. And I want that. I want that.[9]

Many older doctors, in all specialties, are critical of the motivations of younger doctors and students. They perceive them as unwilling to work "hard" enough, or to sacrifice enough. A portion of this is the age-old refrain of older generations about younger; criticizing them for "not being like us." But times have to change, and change is often necessary, in society and in medicine. At one time the old order was slavery, Jim Crow, women not being allowed to vote—younger generations changed this, to the benefit of us all. The old image of the doctor who is always available to his patients must be balanced by the frequent lack of availability that those same doctors had to their families.

Younger doctors wishing to have a more reasonable work-life balance should not be dismissed as simply "lifestyle" issues, but conversely it may be unreasonable to expect the same income as one who works longer hours and is more available. Indeed, current research by the Pew Research Center documented by Paul Taylor in his book *The Next America*, shows that "millennials," people born since 1980 (and thus our medical students and residents), are the most open, accepting, altruistic and optimistic generation alive today. They are optimistic despite the fact that their objective prospects—overall, not just or even maybe including physicians—are worse than those of previous generations.[10] These are, as a generation, outstanding young people and we see many of them in medical schools.

But, of course, we also see the opposite, students whose sole motivation seems to be maximizing income for work, and it is understandable that many older doctors, of any specialty, can find this frustrating. A colleague was very upset about the motivations of some medical students, citing a post from a student on "studentdoctor.net", the largest discussion group for medical students, about whether Allergy should replace Anesthesiology on "the ROAD" (Radiology, Ophthalmology, Anesthesiology, Dermatology, which are widely considered by medical students to be the specialties with the highest income-to-work ratio) because it seemed like "...such a cush job." Then followed a listing of the incomes of different specialists; the low end of all was much higher than the high end of primary care incomes.

But this is the reality. While we are lucky that not all, or even most, medical students are as crass as the student who made the posting above, we cannot ignore the importance of getting equitable reward for work. Some students may be more interested in serving, and be more altruistic and more likely to enter primary care, while others will be more materialistic and self-serving. The latter, I think, should not have gotten into medical school in the first place. They may become interested in primary care, but be unwilling to take an income that is a fraction of that of other specialists. This is the place for public policy.

My colleague commented that "We need a different pool of applicants...We need a different yardstick...We need payment reform. There are plenty of smart people who want to serve. There are a lot of folks who would be thrilled to be the smartest, best paid person in their town." I agree with the sentiment, but it will remain sentiment. It is not an issue of anecdotal preferences of students or doctors. It is a matter of leveling the playing field, or at least reducing the difference. It would be great to have more compassionate, involved caring doctors like Herb Weinman, but our national policy has to be revised so that caring, compassion, availability and hard work are not also associated with the lowest incomes in the house of medicine.

References

1   Chen, C, Petterson, S, Phillips, RL et al., Toward graduate medical education (GME) accountability: measuring the outcomes of GME Institutions, *Acad Med*, 88 (9), September, 2013.

2   *Health Affairs Policy Brief*, Graduate Medical Education, August 31, 2012. http://www.healthaffairs.org/healthpolicybriefs/brief.php?brief_id=75

3   Association of American Medical Colleges. Medicaid graduate medical education payments: A 50-State Survey [Internet]. Washington (DC): *AAMC*, 2013.

4   Ibid #1

5   Ibid #1

6   Ibid #1

7   Freeman J, Petterson, S, Bazemore, A. Accounting for complexity, aligning current payment models with the breadth of care by different specialties. *Amer Fam Phys*, December, 2014.

8   Ibid #1

9   Lewis S, Desperately seeking Herb Weinman, *Pulse*: Voices from the heart of medicine, March 15, 2013. http://pulsemagazine.org/archive/stories/115-desperately-seeking-herb-weinman?highlight=WyJoZXJiIiwid2Vpbm1hbiIsImhlcmIgd2Vpbm1hbiJd

10 Taylor P, and the Pew Research Center. The next America: boomers, millennials, and the looming generational showdown. Public Affairs. New York. 2014.

Chapter 8

Assessing Appropriate Healthcare:
Sometimes the Best Thing is to Do Nothing

Life is not the Land of Oz. You cannot just find the yellow brick road and then follow it, making no further decisions or choices, and know you will get to the Emerald City.

—Anonymous

So far, we have looked at health status in the U.S., compared it to other nations in the developed world, examined the social determinants of health, reviewed the contributions of primary care to the health of the population, and assessed medical school and residency education. In this chapter, I will attempt the treacherous task of trying to help you understand health recommendations, how scientific research progresses, what you see in the latest news that might or might not be important to you, and how to figure that out. I will use some actual health events, reports, and discoveries to illustrate this. I will also try to make clear when there is legitimate controversy. We may say "there are two sides to every story", but in fact often one is right and the other is wrong, especially when the evidence is overwhelming. Finally, I will try to provide some relatively reliable sources of up-to-date information on health care for those who are interested.

In Chapter 6, I discussed the problem of effective communication between doctors and patients, or more generally health care providers and other people. I addressed the need for medical (and other health professions students) to continue to practice communicating in the vernacular even as they learn the new language of "medical" for talking with their peers and teachers. This, alone, is enough cause for confusion.

Another problem challenging people and requiring communication with their health care provider is the onslaught of new information that comes from medical research and frequently makes headlines. Should I get this? Is it good for me? Am I the person for whom this is recommended? Even if I am not, is it still maybe *a little* good for me? What about the fact that I used to hear, and believed, that it was bad for you, and now they are saying it is good? Or, vice versa: that something I thought was good for me is now bad? Why can't they make up their mind? And why do my doctors, or my doctor and my pharmacist, or my doctor and my friend's doctor, or my doctor and my friend/neighbor/relative, disagree?

In this chapter, I will discuss how medical research progresses, why it sometimes seems that something is supposed to be good for you one day and bad for you the next, what influences different recommendations, and how an informed person can think about their own health care.

Sometimes, the number of health recommendations from different sources is so bewildering that it's enough to make you ignore it all. Or, more likely, believe whatever it is you have previously believed. People are very unlikely to change their core beliefs, but even those beliefs that are not so deeply held but have just been around a long time, are resistant to change. If, for years, you've done something based on a belief that it was good for you, or avoided doing something that you believe is bad for you, or if most of your friends think it is good (or bad) for you, and maybe especially if the decision to start doing it was on the advice of a doctor or a big public-health campaign, it is usually going to take more than one news article to change your behavior. In general, this is a good thing—we don't want to keep changing what we do every day—but sometimes there is convincing evidence that demonstrates that we should, and then it isn't such a good idea to hold on. If our beliefs include things like "I don't trust doctors" or "I don't trust science" or "they're always lying to you", it clearly can further complicate our decisions to change or not.

Most of us have someone that we trust for health advice. It could be a doctor or other health professional, one we know in real life or one we see on TV or hear on the radio (hopefully at least a real doctor on an ostensibly real health care show). It could be a friend or relative or neighbor who seems to have some credibility—or a doctor (even if not your own), or nurse, or pharmacist, or *curandera*, or yoga teacher, or neighbor or friend who is just very confident in their beliefs. It is unreasonable to ask of us that we read all the original medical literature, become experts in the understanding and interpretation of it, be able to integrate it into the previously existing literature, and make our health decisions based upon it. Even those who *are* experts, or purport to be, seem to disagree! All of us can get some information from sources on the Internet such as Wikipedia, or search health sites, and this helps, but it is not the same as reading and synthesizing all the primary research on a topic. It is a lot (and probably unreasonable) to expect that even doctors do so.

First, in science and medicine there is very little that is permanent, unchangeable truth. This is different from religion, where faith in core beliefs is often the defining characteristic. As new information is learned, it has to be fit into the information that already exists in order to figure out the most appropriate things to do. When medicine knows something now that is based on the best and newest evidence, and it is different from what we used to believe, this is not a bad thing; it means that science progresses and our understanding is growing. What we knew in the past to be true (provided what we were saying *then* was based on the best evidence available at the time) now must change; what we are certain of now might change when new information becomes available in the future. This is not to be nihilistic, to say "well, then I can never know"; rather, it is to say that what we do and recommend should be based upon the best evidence available at the time.

It is not only pointless, it is often incorrect, to look back and say "Ha! We have been doing what Doctor A said for years, but now it turns out to be wrong! What Doctor B was saying was right all along!" Most of us can recognize the futility of Monday morning quarterbacking, and we need to remember that what seems right now (what Doctor B was "always" advocating) can turn out to be supplanted by new information in the future. I have been in medicine long enough that I can tell stories not only of how "we used to do it, ha ha, how wrong we were", but also of tests and treatment that were right, then wrong, and later right again. In short, what we know shifts over time, and as a patient, you need to do your best to shift with it, recognizing it isn't some lack of principle or shift in integrity, but a constant re-evaluation of what we know and how we know it, that (most of the time) improves things.

Why Do Studies Show Different Things?
How Medical Research Progresses

Science, and scientific research, advances in steps and does not always progress in the same direction. A study is done and it shows a result. It may be good (something is good for you, there is a new treatment that shows promise, there is an old—and cheap—treatment that works as well or better than a new, expensive one) or bad (a test or treatment that is widespread is ineffective or even harmful, something in the environment or our food is bad for our health). This is not the end, though, even when the research is of high quality. One of the characteristics of most scientific research is that it tries, to the extent possible, to control all variables but one as a way of seeing if that one made a difference. Think of a trial of a new treatment for a disease. Researchers will want the study subjects who take the treatment and those who don't to be as similar as possible, to not have any significantly different health practices or other diseases; they don't want to have one group have disease in a more advanced stage, or to have all men or women, or African-Americans or Euro-Americans, or old people or young people, in one group. They then *randomize* people to either receive treatment or not so that any difference that they didn't think of (say, whether people do yoga or not) is as likely to be present in one group as another. They don't tell people whether they are getting the treatment or not (called a blinded study), and who is getting the treatment is also unknown to the researchers assessing the effect (double-blinded). This sort of test, a double-blinded *randomized controlled trial (RCT),* is considered the gold standard of medical research. In evaluating treatments, this is really the only kind of study that can be relied on.

But even this "gold standard" test has its limitations, and so not everything can be tested with RCTs. For one thing, an RCT is only good for answering some kinds of questions, mainly regarding treatment. Other important types of studies include choosing the best diagnostic test, evaluating the natural history of a disease, or trying to figure out *why* something is happening—especially with regard to human behavior. These involve different types of studies.*A new test is usually compared to the best test currently available. We look to see if the new test is more accurate, less dangerous, or cheaper than the current one.[1]

Another concern with RCTs is that one of their defining characteristics is the attempt to control for most things other than the question under study. This may mean that it is not certain whether the results will apply to people whose lives are not so tightly controlled—that is, most of us. This is why science requires that not only the results, but the methods, selection criteria and the processes followed in a research study be publicly available. This allows others to replicate the studies to ensure that they find the same results, or change the study somewhat to find out if it works the same way in a different group of people. Often, later studies will show different results from the first ones, and this also adds to our sum of knowledge and can elucidate what the reasons for the differences were. RCTs are expensive, difficult and time consuming, especially when the outcome being examined is something as definitive as death or serious suffering. This means that sometimes the findings of one study will govern our behavior for a long time before another is done.

*A good resource: Sackett, DL, *Clinical Epidemiology : A Basic Science For Clinical Medicine, 2nd Ed.* Little, Brown. Boston. 1991.

Furthermore, human biology is very complex, with changes in one area often having a significant impact elsewhere. The simple answer we would like, "if I do this, it is good, and if I do more of it, that will be better" (or the opposite, "the less of this I do the better"), is rarely true. Even the concept of "do things in moderation" is not always true, although it is often closer to the best idea than the extremes. Life, a wise person once said, is not the Land of Oz. You cannot just find the yellow brick road and then follow it, making no further decisions or choices, and know you will get to the Emerald City. Of course, this was not even true in the Land of Oz; there were obstacles along the way and the Wonderful Wizard was a charlatan. There are, however, a few areas where we have enough knowledge. There is no "good" or even not-harmful amount of cigarette smoking; in this area we have definitive evidence that any amount of smoking, even that received second-hand, is bad for your health.[2]

Guidelines, Bias, and Your Health

The massive, and growing body of information about diseases, diagnoses, and especially treatments that is available is one of the challenges in educating health-care professionals, students and residents, and in continuing education. If a doctor or nurse or pharmacist knows only what they learned in school, it will be outdated in a very few years. Thus, the health professions have committed to the concept of "life-long learning," but ensuring that it is effective and accurate is an ongoing challenge.

With the development of the Internet, information is widely shared very quickly, and this information is available not only to health professionals but to everyone. In the "old days", someone with symptoms, or a new diagnosis, might go to the library, or find a copy of Morris Fishbein's *Handy Home Medical Encyclopedia.* Now they go to the Internet and are overwhelmed with information. The problem is that this information may be correct, partially correct, or totally wrong. It may be complete, incomplete, or valueless. There is a difference between information and truth, and certainly between information and wisdom. Wisdom and truth require information, but much available information is chaff, or worse. It is important to find reliable sources of information: often, in medicine, these are sites run by well-known universities or providers, including Harvard, Johns Hopkins, and the Mayo Clinic. It is also important to find ways to check on whether something you read is supported by evidence, especially if the information seems to be too good to be true, by looking at several independent sources.

If keeping up with information and sifting through it to discover what is true, relevant, and important is hard for a person who wants to find out about their one condition, it is truly daunting for health professionals who need to keep up on many. There are so many drugs! And new ones all the time! And they are all "better, improved, and more effective" (and certainly more expensive) than the old ones. Until, of course, we find out that they are not. Or, worse, they are dangerous. Sometimes they are so dangerous that they have to be pulled from the market. How can health professionals avoid being completely overwhelmed and paralyzed by trying to get through this mass of "information" to "truth"? Jerry Avorn, a very highly regarded physician, considers this situation to be an example of Stendhal Syndrome, named after the writer who experienced serious physical symptoms after seeing the surfeit of great art in Florence in 1817.[3] How can we most effectively help, and *primum non nocere,* first do no harm?

One traditional method, adopted by our friends in the drug industry, has been "detailing." Pharmaceutical representatives (called, regardless of gender, "detail men") fanned out, visiting physicians, giving out free samples of their wares as well as food and pens and sticky-note pads and clocks and calendars and little scale models of whatever organ their drug worked on, along with information about the drug. The information might have been accurate and complete, but often was skewed to make the drug look as good as possible, and often based upon research funded by the manufacturer (as opposed to the government, through the National Institutes of Health (NIH), or other agencies, or independent foundations). The detail men were easily identifiable, even when not pushing a cart full of pizza for "grand rounds" because they were all good-looking and so much more well-dressed than run-of-the-mill health care workers. What a great system! You get information about new drugs, direct from the person selling them, and little scale models of the urinary system, complete with donuts too! Isn't that how we all hoped our doctors were keeping up with the information they need to care for our health? Ethics rules have since limited the ubiquity of detail men, free gifts, and even samples. The "educational cruises" to the Caribbean for being a high utilizer of a company's drugs are all but gone. Avorn describes a much more insidious effort, however—the influence that these companies have on the development of "clinical guidelines" that recommend how drugs should be prescribed to patients by groups of experts in a particular medical field.

Given the information glut, clinical guidelines are critical. Sifting through all the data is almost impossible to do for all the conditions that exist, especially ones that are seen rarely by a particular practitioner. It makes sense that a group of experts in the field review all the evidence in that narrow area and make recommendations that we can count on to be accurate and can utilize effectively. But we may be reaching a point where there are too many guidelines, often with conflicting recommendations. Avorn's discussion of recommendations from the American Association of Clinical Endocrinologists (AACE) on caring for patients with diabetes is fairly damning in this respect; he notes that they:

> ... *elevate many second- or third-line drugs to more prominent positions in the prescribing hierarchy, rivaling once uncontested go-to medications like metformin, an inexpensive generic. They also emphasize the riskiness of established treatments like insulin and glipizide, which now carry yellow warning labels... Several of the now promoted drugs are expensive newcomers that lack the track records of clinical effectiveness and safety held by the older, potentially displaced treatments... the manufacturers of some of these new drugs financially supported the development of the guidelines, and many of the authors are paid consultants to some of those companies.*[4]

In addition to citing previous examples of expert-generated and industry-sponsored guidelines that have led to overuse of drugs with very bad outcomes for patients, Avorn also cites reliable sources of clinical guidelines, based solely on review of the evidence, not the opinions of experts that might be influenced by money. The sources he suggests include the Institute of Medicine, the American College of Physicians, and the Cochrane Collaboration (an international network of experts that evaluates clinical research). These are the kinds of sources from which your doctor should be getting information.

There are at least two other sources of bias beyond any direct influence exerted by drug company funding of research, guidelines development, and individual experts. One is the fact that many treatments, particularly when they involve procedures, can increase the income of the individual physicians doing them and the revenues of the hospitals in which they work. This may be the reason that many procedures have been and continue to be done, for which the evidence supporting their effectiveness is weak. One example may be in the stent placed in the heart of former President George W. Bush, an intervention that was not necessary based on evidence available to the public. President Bush had a "routine annual physical" which included a cardiac stress test that led to a CT angiogram that found a blockage that led to the placement of a stent. The problem is that a stent in an artery does not prevent progression of disease, although it can relieve pain. But the President didn't have pain; as noted by in the *New York Times* by Prasad and Cifu:

Before he underwent his annual physical, Mr. Bush reportedly had no symptoms. Quite the opposite: His exercise tolerance was astonishing for his age, 67. He rode more than 30 miles in the heat on a bike ride for veterans injured in the wars in Iraq and Afghanistan.[5]

In this particular case, money may not have been the motivator as much as "do everything" for the former President, but the result is that many other people will feel that inappropriate testing and treatment, if OK for President Bush, is good for them (and that they are being cheated if they do not get it).

As a result of different perspectives and indeed conflicts of interest, guidelines issued by different organizations can be in conflict. An excellent example is mammographic screening for breast cancer, enormously controversial because of the high profile of this disease, the lack of any known prevention, and the large and well-funded advocacy community. In a 2013 article in *JAMA,* Michael Marmot addresses the potential benefits and harms from different guidelines, focusing on UK recommendations,[6] and Kachalia and Mello examine the differing U.S. recommendations from the U.S. Preventive Services Task Force (USPSTF), American Cancer Society (ACS), and American College of Radiology (ACR).[7] If a radiologist reads a mammogram as normal, but, following ACR guidelines, recommends another in one year, while the clinician is following USPSTF guidelines for less frequent screening, does that place the clinician at increased legal risk? They argue at least for consistent guidelines to be utilized within a single institution.

Finally, there is the potential for unintended outcomes. One of the most reliable evidence-based sources of recommendations is the U.S. Preventive Services Task Force (USPSTF). Its recommendations are based solely on review of the science, which has generated controversy when those recommendations were unpopular with powerful groups. For example, a major review of 30 years of mammography screening was published in the *New England Journal of Medicine* in 2012, which found that screening mammograms have uncovered a large number of early-stage breast cancers; in fact, over that time, the number of early-stage breast cancers identified had doubled (from 112 to 234 cases per 100,000 women per year).[8] This would be a good thing, if these cancers can be treated and prevent women from dying or suffering serious morbidity. If in fact this were happening, then (assuming the actual rate of cancer stays the same) the number of cancers diagnosed in later stages, where intervention is less successful, should go down. That is, those cancers detected early and treated would not progress and should mean that many fewer women present with later stage cancer.

Unfortunately, the study demonstrated that this has not occurred. The decrease in late-stage cancer diagnosis has been about 8 per 100,000 women per year. So, for every 100,000 women, we are diagnosing an additional 122 early stage cancers, but only decreasing the number of late stage cancers by 8. Because, as doctors and scientists know, not all cancer progresses—some (maybe most) resolve by themselves before becoming a problem—this means that most of the additional women found by mammography to have early stage breast cancer would not have progressed to late-stage cancer. Thus they assert, with good reason, that cancer was over-diagnosed—in 70,000 women in 2008 alone. Any estimate of the number of lives saved by screening and early intervention is inflated if it includes large numbers of women whose cancers would not have progressed. In other words, many of these women diagnosed with cancer, many of whom had non-trivial interventions (surgery, radiation, chemotherapy) had cancers that would, basically, have not required any treatment.[9] In responding to the study, some radiologists who do mammograms said that the findings were "junk science." This is not a reasonable response to a well-done piece of research that reaches conclusions you don't like.

However, reliance on science does not obviate the "law of unintended consequences." The reliability of recommendations from the USPSTF, and the fact that they are based in science, led them to be written into the health reform law, the ACA, which mandates insurers pay for preventive services with an "A" or "B" recommendation from USPSTF. However, as articulately described by USPSTF members Steven Woolf and Doug Campos-Outcalt,[10] this creates the unintended consequence of turning USPSTF into a group that effectively decides whether companies and doctors will make money; you can imagine the lobbying by a company to try to prove that its product deserves a "B" rating!

Rationing, Waste, and Useless Interventions

When people themselves, or those they love, are sick, they want things done for them that might be of benefit. Cost may be a secondary factor, especially when it is not directly being borne by them because they have good health insurance. The order of preference would presumably be for:

1. Things that will definitely help;
2. Things that might help;
3. Things that almost certainly won't help but-you-never-know and don't cause serious harm; and
4. Avoid things that won't help and may very well cause serious harm.

While it might seem that you wouldn't want interventions in that last group, people do opt for them. This is particularly common when the expected outcome is death; if you're going to die anyway, what harm could be greater? Besides, maybe a miracle will occur. The problem is that there can be greater harm than simply dying: death preceded by increased suffering caused by futile attempts at treatment is a step backward, not forward. But instead of confronting death, many people look at the positives of a treatment and ignore the negatives.

There are also powerful cultural norms that urge people on to more treatment, as if this is a war. People "do battle" with cancer, they die "after a long fight", they die after "losing the fight." In this context, a choice to discontinue treatment is like admitting defeat, like quitting, being a loser. It's no wonder, then, with these metaphors combined with a desperate hope against hope that people "soldier" on, bravely trying one last thing.

But whether someone survives cancer is less about winning a war than it is about how old the person is, being lucky, privileged, having early intervention, and other complicating factors. Those things, plus effective tools at the disposal of the doctor. When the tools are very effective, we drop the war metaphors. No one speaks of "winning their battle" against appendicitis. Everyone recognizes that the determining factor was not the patient's resolve but the luck of getting to the hospital on time plus the doctor's great tools. We say, "I had my appendix out." One day, if the tools get good enough, we might say, "I got my cancer out." But today, we get confused about the role resolve plays because the tools for fighting cancer, some cancers anyway, are so poor.

While we wait for the day that those tools and cures arrive, we need care and wisdom in choosing the treatments that are available, recognizing their power, limits, and harm, and that these exist independent of the patient's will to live. In addition, the decision may be different when it is made by the person actually facing death (provided s/he is conscious and competent—or has advance directives) from when it is made by others, including his/her loved ones.

The real problem is that the expense of our health system is enormous and some, or much, of that spending is on diagnostic tests that may not alter treatment or treatments that may not offer much, or any, benefit. How much potential benefit must there be for an intervention to be worth its cost? Obviously, this depends on the cost, but it also depends upon who it is for. If it is for *me* I might have a different answer than if it is for someone I don't know. And even if it is for me, I might have a different answer if I am paying out of my own pocket or if my insurance is paying for it. Ultimately, however, we all pay for treatment, either out of our pockets, out of our insurance premiums or out of our tax dollars. Having a rational approach would be useful.

Am I suggesting rationing of health care? Yes, but more importantly I am suggesting that health care is already rationed, but that the criteria by which it is rationed are not always explicit. In general, people with good insurance and money get things done to them, even when those things may not be really beneficial, while others do not always get care that we know to be of benefit. An equitable and just health care system can be consistent with rationing provided that the criteria for doing so are based on the person's illness and probability of benefit, rather than the person's wealth and probability of profit for those doing the intervening.

What about the rationing of health resources? Howard Brody, a medical ethicist, writes;

First, rationing occurs simply because resources are finite and someone must decide who gets what. Second, rationing is therefore inevitable; if we avoid explicit rationing, we will resort to implicit and perhaps unfair rationing methods. The main ethical objection to rationing is that physicians owe an absolute duty of fidelity to each individual patient, regardless of cost. This objection fails, however, because when re-

sources are exhausted, the patients who are deprived of care are real people and not statistics. Physicians collectively owe loyalty to those patients too.[11]

This is an excellent example of the key principle of "justice" in medical ethics. From the viewpoint of social justice, while Brody is writing in the abstract, we need only look around at what is actually occurring in the world to know that we have rationing that is unfair. Of course, some resources are more limited than others. Most other countries, with better health status, are able to provide the most useful care because they don't spend money providing worthless care. In the U.S., one of the main efforts to control costs has been to limit the duration of hospitalizations, and to do many things on an outpatient basis that used to be done in hospitals. In many other developed countries, however, hospitalization rates are higher and length of stay is longer, but costs are lower? How come?

The most important difference is in the cost of interventions, especially high-tech interventions, in this country. It is possible to have someone in the hospital (as they do in other places) for relatively longer stays, getting relatively low-cost care, the kind that in the U.S. usually will not "qualify" for hospitalization. On the other hand, it is possible to have a very short stay in which many tests and interventions are done and the cost is very high. The principles of equity and justice do not require that everyone receive the *same* care, but that they receive the care they need. Consider two people with the same condition, say pneumonia. One lives in a nice house, and has family to care for him, prepare food, ensure that he gets his medication. The other has no family and is homeless, has no way to ensure that he has food, warmth, or even shelter, and no place to store medications. It might be perfectly reasonable for the first person to be treated at home; indeed, most of us in such a situation would prefer it. But it might be appropriate for the second person to remain in the hospital for a much longer time for treatment. To not do so could easily result in his getting sicker, being re-admitted, and maybe dying. The same treatment is not right for both people.

Brody notes that of the 30% of medical expenditures that are "waste", only about 10% are due to deliberate fraud. This is far too much fraud, but doing unnecessary things because they make money is more than just "waste", it is irresponsible and unjust. So while eliminating fraud is important, it is a "one-time" saving, whereas eliminating waste not only represents a bigger number, but, because doing more and more tests is a major driver of rising health costs, may represent a way to "bend the cost curve." Of course, what is "waste" can depend upon one's perspective, values, and even degree of selfishness. Because one person's health expense (even if it is "waste") is another person's income, this becomes a complex political discussion.

Brody cites the case of treatment of advanced metastatic breast cancer with high-dose chemotherapy followed by autologous* bone marrow transplantation, which was:

...initially thought to offer perhaps a 10% chance of a significant extension of life for patients who would otherwise be fated to die very soon. Insurers' refusal to pay the high

---

* This means that they take out a piece of your bone marrow (which produces blood cells), before giving you radiation that will destroy your marrow, and then transplant the piece back into you.

costs of this last-chance treatment did much to torpedo pub-lic trust in managed care during the 1990s. Data now sug-gest that the actual chance of meaningful benefit from this treatment is zero and that the only effect of the treatment was to make patients' remaining months of life miserable.[12]

Yes, it could have gone the other way; maybe longer experi-ence would have shown it to be more effective. As I have argued previously, we have to make decisions based on the best data we have at the time, whatever we may later learn. However, in this case the best data at the time did not show that there was a benefit, as there was insufficient evidence to know if it was of benefit or not. In this setting, the assumption by many was that "doing some-thing" was better than doing nothing. The managed care compa-nies that initially refused to pay for unproven treatment were vili-fied both by advocacy groups and from physicians and hospitals that benefited financially from these procedures. The result, as it turned out, was patients suffered with no real chance of benefit.

Is debunking ineffective screening and therapy removing hope or just removing risk?

I am a doctor; I want to help people, to relieve their suffer-ing, to help facilitate the cure of their diseases when possible. More than that, I am a family doctor, and have a strong prefer-ence for prevention, for early detection of disease when it is still treatable rather than waiting for it to be too far gone for treatment to be effective. In addition, I have regularly criticized our health system for leaving out too many people, creating financial disin-centives for them to seek care early. This leads to their waiting until their diseases become so uncontrolled that they present to the emergency room, then require hospital admission and costly care, making it worse for them and more expensive for everyone. So I think prevention and early intervention is a really good thing, and it is great when we have tests that can identify disease early in its course so that we can change its trajectory.

But because I want these things to be true doesn't make them true. While I do not wish to sound like a medical nihilist, there are many places in medicine where a diagnostic test, a treatment, or even a preventive screening test promises more than it can deliver. Because we can screen you for something doesn't mean that we should; because a test can be done doesn't mean that it is a good test. "A good test", in my opinion, is one that has sufficient sensitivity (rate of being positive when a condition is present) and specificity (rate of being negative when a condition is absent) to tell us with sufficient likelihood that you have a disease (or don't), or if it matters. Because a test can be done also doesn't mean that it is cost-effective or even worthwhile. Because a treatment exists doesn't mean it is a good treatment, a safe treatment, an effective treatment. And, as with most things being sold, the greater the publicity and advertising around it, the more it means someone will be making money on it. This does not exclude the possibility of its being of benefit, but is certainly not the same thing.

Sometimes, when evidence is discovered that a test or treatment is not of benefit, we eventually stop doing it. "Eventually", however, may be a lot longer than you might think. In a 2012 *JAMA* article, Prasad, Cifu, and Ionannidis note that:

Ideally, good medical practices are replaced by better ones, based on robust comparative trials in which new interven-

tions outperform older ones and establish new standards of care. Often, however, established standards must be abandoned not because a better replacement has been identified but simply because what was thought to be beneficial was not.[13]

They go on to discuss a number of treatments that have been "standard of care" but were shown by good randomized controlled trials to be ineffective or even dangerous, not to mention expensive. These include stenting of coronary arteries for stable coronary artery disease (CAD), postmenopausal hormone therapy to prevent CAD, vertebroplasty for osteoporotic fractures, bevucizamab for breast cancer. Unsurprisingly, "true believers" continued to defend these interventions even after the evidence was clear (perhaps because their livelihoods depend upon it), and in many cases these treatments continue to be offered and performed.

There are thousands of clinical trials, but most deal with trivialities or efforts to buttress the sales of specific products. Rarely, some investigators find the courage to test established "truths" with large, rigorous randomized trials. Indeed, Prasad and colleagues have done many of these latter trials; John Ioannidis is the "guru" of debunking treatments with poor evidence. [14]

Prevention and screening are also subject to the lure of magical thinking compounded by the greed of the sellers. Screening for prostate cancer with the use of prostate-specific antigen (PSA) testing is an example. It was widely promoted for years as a screening test for prostate cancer, despite being poorly sensitive (a lot of people who had cancer had normal PSAs) and poorly specific (a lot of people with high PSAs did not have cancer). When the U.S. Preventive Services Task Force (USPSTF) first recommended that men over a certain age no longer be screened, and later when they finally recommended against all PSA screening, there was a strong backlash, especially from urologists. But now even urologists recognize that not all men should be screened, although they still have laxer criteria than the USPSTF.

Prostate cancer is one of those cancers that can be very aggressive, metastasize, and kill someone painfully, but most of the time is something incidentally found at autopsy; in these cases it is a disease people "die with" rather than "die from." PSAs cannot tell the difference, so doing them leads to further testing, which can have its own morbidity as well as cost (ultrasounds and biopsies) and often lead to treatment with serious cost and morbidity (incontinence, impotence, radiation effects) even though the disease may have never manifested itself. Moreover, there is very weak evidence that treatment of any kind alters the course of the disease in most cases; those who have the "bad" kind of prostate cancer usually die despite treatment and those who have the "good" kind live with or without treatment. It would be great if we had a test you could get that would be better able to tell us if you had the "bad" kind of prostate cancer, and even better if we could prevent the progression of the "bad" kind without unnecessarily treating those with the "good" kind and causing serious morbidity. But because it would be good if we had it, we do not yet.

Another example is the annual pelvic exam. Here we are not talking about the Pap smear for cervical cancer (which is not recommended annually), but the part where the doctor puts her/his hands inside for an exam. In the absence of any symptoms (pain, discharge, bleeding) the pelvic exam is by definition a screening test. However, there is no evidence at all that there is any disease for which it is an effective screen (for example, ovarian cancer cannot be detected by this method until it is very advanced). As noted in a recent *New York Times* editorial, "The Dispute Over Annual Pelvic Exams," the American College of Physicians (internists) now recommends against it[15], but the American College of Obstetricians and Gynecologists (ACOG) continues to defend it. Indeed, the reasons put forward by ACOG quoted in the editorial range from the indefensible (that it is good even though it is not evidence based) to the absurd (that it is the way to find problems like incontinence and sexual dysfunction):

...the gynecologists group argues that the "clinical experiences" of gynecologists, while not "evidence-based," demonstrate that annual pelvic exams are useful in detecting problems like incontinence and sexual dysfunction and in establishing a dialogue with patients about a wide range of health issues.[16]

If a woman has incontinence or sexual dysfunction, she knows it and the way to discover it is not by a pelvic exam, but by asking her! Obviously, this is also the way to establish a dialogue about a wide range of health issues.

Pap smears are fairly good screening tests for cervical cancer, but most other cancer screening tests (even mammograms and colon cancer screening, probably the next best) are not nearly as good. Every time there is a recommendation to decrease the frequency of screening (Pap smears, mammography) or not do them at all (PSAs or pelvic exams), there is an outcry from people who think that something has been taken from them. In a scientific sense, what has been taken is unnecessary testing that doesn't lower their risk of bad outcomes, costs money, and can have significant morbidity when false-positive screening tests lead to additional, more invasive tests. But, in a more metaphysical sense, when a test that has been used is found to be of little value, we may take away peoples' hope—the idea that there is something that they can do that will prevent something bad from happening to them. The test is viewed as something that, while perhaps a little risky, is relatively easy. And also, frankly, something that someone else can do, rather than something hard that you yourself have to do, like, say, dieting or giving up smoking or exercising. Far easier to take a test. And this false hope is encouraged by half-truths promulgated by passionate advocates of interventions with limited proven benefit, whether traditional or "alternative."

The "Choosing Wisely" Campaign:
Sometimes the Best Thing to Do is Nothing

In an effort to get physicians to make better decisions about the tests and treatments that they order, the American Board of Internal Medicine (ABIM) Foundation has developed an initiative called *Choosing Wisely* that calls on medical specialty societies to list 5 tests or treatments frequently performed in their specialty that they recommend not be done, or not be done on most patients.[17] As of this writing there are 53 societies that have lists, some with more than 5 items. The list of the American Academy of Family Physicians (AAFP), for example, now includes 15 items.

Soon after the initiative commenced in 2012, I was interviewed by a radio talk show host, who had questions about some of the recommendations. For example, one of the recommendations from the American Society of Clinical Oncologists' (ASCO) is:

Don't use cancer-directed therapy for solid tumor patients with the following characteristics: low performance status (3 or 4), no benefit from prior evidence-based interventions, not eligible for a clinical trial, and no strong evidence supporting the clinical value of further anticancer treatment. [18]

This basically says "don't use dangerous treatments that don't work." I figured it for a no-brainer, but the host asked, "What if a patient wants treatment for cancer anyway?" I said I thought it was the responsibility of the doctor to point out that the treatment would not help, and would not only cost money but would have a lot of toxic side effects; I said that I thought that most people, if they knew they were going to die from their cancer and the treatment would not help, would not wish to spend their last days and weeks nauseated, losing their hair, and being unable to interact comfortably with their loved ones. Was he satisfied? I don't know. Would you be? It was my best effort at the time.

Each "choosing wisely" recommendation that a test or treatment *not* be performed is backed by the evidence, and is accompanied by a summary of the reasons. One of the recommendations from the AAFP is "Don't routinely prescribe antibiotics for acute mild-to-moderate sinusitis unless symptoms last for seven or more days, or symptoms worsen after initial clinical improvement," and the evidence summary says:

Most sinusitis in the ambulatory setting is due to a viral infection that will resolve on its own. Despite consistent recommendations to the contrary, antibiotics are prescribed in more than 80% of outpatient visits for acute sinusitis. Sinusitis accounts for 16 million office visits and $5.8 billion in annual health care costs. [19]

That is big money for a treatment that doesn't work, and can cause bad side effects (allergies to the antibiotics and increased resistance of bacteria to antibiotics, for example). It would be even better if the money not spent were available to meet the real health needs of those who need it most.

The radio host said "We are always being told patients should be self-advocates. What if in advocating for ourselves we say we want antibiotics for our sinusitis?"

His comments may not have been meant to be provocative, but it is a good question, illustrating the pressure that health care providers are under to do something even when they know nothing will have a positive impact. It also illustrates the success that patient advocacy movements have had in increasing the awareness of people that they should be involved in their own health care decisions. However, this is not the same as going into a grocery store and buying whatever you want. It is the responsibility of the medical provider to supply the options and recommendations for a patient to choose from but not to simply provide anything the patient wants.

It is important to note that there are two very different kinds of recommendations that can be made br campaigns such as "Choosing Wisely" or by other sources. One advises that things be done differently—use medicines better, admit more service minded medical students, and so on. The other is actually redesigning the system: make it illegal or not pay for antibiotics for sinusitis, abandon fee for service payments, raise the pay of PCPs. The first set will have a limited impact. The second set represents redesigning the system for different outcomes. Which set is more important? It's very important not to split the difference. Yes, the first set can help, just as bed rest can be good for a patient with appendicitis. But real interventions are needed—and are quite different.

Health economists often note that the reason why people may demand unnecessary diagnostic tests and useless treatments is that they expect them to be covered by their health insurance, that they have no "skin in the game." This is likely to be in part true. There are many things that a patient might want, legitimately or not (prescription drugs, disabled parking stickers, diagnostic tests), that can only be obtained with a physician's approval. But even people with no insurance and little money still want "the best" for themselves and their loved ones, and they in particular may feel that the reason it is being denied is that they are poor. However, the problem of wasteful medicine is not confined to those with great insurance.

Decades ago, when Woody Allen was a standup comic, he did a famous bit in which he complains of pain in the "chestal area." He is pretty sure it is heartburn, but is worried and doesn't want to pay the $25 to see a doctor (it was a long time ago). Luckily his friend, Eggs Benedict, is having the same kind of pain, and he figures if he can get Eggs to go to the doctor, he can find out what it is and save money. It works, and Eggs finds out it is heartburn. Two days later, he discovers Eggs is dead. He immediately checks into the hospital, has all kinds of tests, and discovered he has—heartburn. The bill is $110 (it was a really long time ago). He goes to see Eggs' mother and asks if his friend suffered much. "No," she says, "the car hit him and that was it!"[20]

In the opening chapter, I discussed the 4 key principles of medical ethics: beneficence (do good), non-maleficence (do no harm), autonomy, and justice. The same week as the radio interview, I facilitated a discussion about futile treatment at the end of life for a group of third-year medical students in their medical ethics course. They had just received a lecture from a distinguished medical oncologist, who had presented the four core principles of medical ethics. They also read several articles documenting cases in which end of life decision-making did not go smoothly or well, and the article *How Doctors Die* by Ken Murray.[21] One of the cases involved a patient with terminal cancer who had already failed treatment, and for whom further treatment would be futile and have adverse effects. He had agreed to hospice, and to comfort care, until a relative (a physician!) came to town and demanded additional treatment for him, and convinced the patient to demand it as well. The medical students, who had all been through clinical experiences and most of whom had been part of teams that confronted dealing effectively with dying patients, were in agreement with the physician in the article, and with each other, that the treatment was futile and would be a bad idea. However, several felt that, if the patient demanded it, the principle of autonomy required that it be given. Others noted that this might violate the principle of non-maleficence. I pointed out that that there were many areas in which we do not allow the patient to pick his/her treatment of choice. For example, we do not allow people to walk into a pharmacy and buy narcotic pain relievers without a prescription, no matter how much they might want them. And doctors are increasingly held to account when they over prescribe narcotics. Certainly the effects of chemotherapy poisons were at least as great.

Thus these core principles of medical ethics do not exist in isolation; they interact with each other. As discussed earlier, I noted that I believe that justice is least discussed and least understood, but that, at its core, it is about people with the same conditions having the same options. This does not explicitly mean that a person should not have a treatment that will do them no good and may do them harm, but it does mean that in a society with limited resources (and all societies have limited resources), unnecessary or dangerous treatments delivered to some people limit the options for others, or, at least, would if the money for health care were held in common, and savings in one area could be used to address needs in another.

Of course, this is more the case the more limited a society's resources are, and also how widely (equitably, justly) the benefits are distributed. In some poor countries which have undergone change (electoral or revolutionary) that sought to create greater equality, goods that were not seen by the privileged to be scarce before (say milk, shoes) suddenly became more scarce when they were now being distributed to everyone. In our own society, the big challenge is that savings from not delivering inappropriate care to some will not be used to deliver appropriate care to others, but rather only to increase insurance company profit. This, of course, is why a rational system of distributing care requires an equitable system of paying for it.

These are not always easy decisions, but it is one of the reasons being a doctor is hard, respected, and (at least relatively) well-paid. If everything were a simple algorithm and one could just memorize the right answer as these medical students were expected to do so often on their multiple-choice tests, it could be done by someone with much less training. And, to be fair, they are often decisions that doctors are reluctant to make; they often opt to do more even when it is unlikely to help a person because deciding not to is hard. The area of palliative care and hospice care is one place where such decisions are being actively considered, and we can expect that, as the hospice movement and end of life palliative care training of physicians improves, so will these decisions.

Sure, it is possible for someone getting antibiotics for viral sinusitis to get better—indeed they usually do, with or without the antibiotics. Temporal association is not cause. Thus, even when you do the right thing, based on the evidence, and do not get a test or treatment, it is still possible that you will end up worse—as Eggs and Woody discovered.

Patient-Centered Research vs Disease-Centered Research: Answering the Questions That Matter to People

It would make sense to most people that medical research should be focused, at least in large part, on answering the questions that matter to people. The Methodology Committee of the Patient Centered Outcomes Research Institute (PCORI), a government supported center created by the ACA to sponsor research with patient-centered outcomes, writes that:

Large investments are too often made in studies that provide poor-quality evidence, are overtly biased, are not applicable to most patients, or yield results that do not address the real concerns of individuals facing clinical decisions.[23]

Indeed, this is in fact characteristic of *most* research, whether sponsored by the National Institutes of Health (NIH), foundations, or private companies. The reasons for this are that such research is easier to do and relatively well-funded (the "large investments"). Of course, much research is, and should be, very basic, looking at the mechanisms of human biology and discovering information that *may,* someday, be the useful basis for answering questions that matter to people. But this is not what the PCORI group is addressing. They are talking about research at the clinical level, research that, even if not of poor quality or overtly biased, does not yield results important to people as it is not designed to do so.

One important concept (initially identified mainly by primary care researchers) distinguishes between "disease-oriented evidence" (DOE) and "patient-oriented evidence" (POE, or later, adding "that matters", POEM). The first focuses on the disease: such research might show that a treatment combats the disease. The second looks at what treatments improve the life of a person. There is a big difference. An example might be research to discover a regimen for diabetes that minimizes the complications from high blood sugar by keeping the average blood sugar much lower than had previously been the goal (called "tight control"). Disease-oriented evidence might show that using frequent insulin injections to keep the blood sugar in the low-normal range reduces the long-term negative effects of diabetes. A patient-oriented approach, however, looks at the overall impact on the person, not just the disease. Does the patient find it difficult to administer more frequent injections of insulin and check their blood sugar? If they do injections more frequently, do they spend a significant amount of time with blood sugar that is in fact too low (after all, reducing the *average* increases the probability that sometimes it will be too low), and feel fuzzy-headed and unable to live the lives they wish to? Or feel dizzy? Or that a certain percent actually pass out from low blood sugar? Do more patients break their hips and end up in the hospital and even die from its complications? Can this happen even though their diabetes is in "good" control? I am reminded of a famous saying. "The disease was controlled but the patient died from a complication of treatment." This is not a desirable patient-oriented outcome.

The motivation for private companies, most often pharmaceutical companies, to fund disease-oriented research is fairly obvious. Their sole agenda is to make a profit, so they are interested in supporting research that shows that their drugs are effective for treating certain conditions. They have a number of advantages in this arena:

- Showing "effectiveness" requires, by Food and Drug Administration (FDA) criteria, only to show that a new drug or other treatment is more effective than a placebo, not more effective than currently available treatments;
- Since they are paying for it, they can suppress the publication of results that do not show their drugs in a good light, leaving only the good stories in the picture;
- They have to show only that it modifies the disease, not that it is the best choice for any individual patient (thus it is *disease*-oriented, rather than *patient*-oriented);
- In lieu of patient-centered research, they have huge marketing budgets (far in excess of their research budgets) to advertise their products to both providers and directly to patients once they have been approved by the FDA.
- Patient-centered research might lead to less profitable outcomes, if it shows that a treatment that might make the disease better actually makes the patient worse.

The reasons that the NIH would mostly fund this sort of research are complicated. A big part of it is, simply, that is what researchers do. An entire industry has been built around doing disease-oriented research, both in biological science laboratories and clinical trials in people. Thousands of academics and the institutions at which they work are dependent upon such funding to maintain and advance their careers and institutions. The review committees that make recommendations to approve or disapprove funding are "peer" committees, made up of people who do, largely, the same kind of work. This is good because they can understand and evaluate the science involved (a really *bad* thing would be for a group of politically-appointed ideologues to make the decisions, and this sometimes has occurred), but they may be limited by their preconceived notions of how "good" research is done and, more important, what its goals should be.

This relates to a second challenge—patient-oriented research is more complicated, more difficult to do, and leads to less "clear" outcomes. Of course, it is more relevant to patients and their providers making decisions about their care, but it is harder to fit into a rigid research model in which all but one variable is tightly controlled. This can lead to research that is done because it is possible to do it, rather than because it answers the questions that we might have. Most traditional NIH researchers have no objection to patient-oriented research, but in an era of limited funding availability, they might be quite concerned if funding it decreased the amount available for the kind of work that they do.

The establishment of PCORI by the ACA was intended to apply the rigorous standards of Clinical Effectiveness Research (CER) to the treatment of *patients,* not diseases. One reason, which should be obvious, is that people, particularly older people, often have more than one disease. The "right" treatment for a patient's cancer needs to take into account its effect on his/her other condition(s): diabetes—or heart disease, hypertension, arthritis, depression, alcoholism, glaucoma, poverty, and yes, maybe, an-other cancer—in any or all combinations.

Outcomes That Matter To Patients

In deciding how much attention to give research results, it is clearly critical to look at the outcomes being measured. The concept of patient-oriented evidence (POE) vs. disease-oriented evidence (DOE) is one consideration, but ultimately we should be concerned with only patient-*important* outcomes. There are only two negative ones: premature death and reduced quality of life, or in positive terms, greater longevity and better quality of life. Some research looks at these outcomes, but it is not always fea-sible. Death is a one-time-per-person event, and everyone dies, so using this as an outcome measure requires a lot of people and a long time. Quality of life has, in some sense, the opposite prob-lem in that it changes often, and can be the result of many factors, thus making it difficult to measure. So, studies measuring the two patient-important outcomes are quite rare. For example, Gandhi and colleagues reviewed all the randomized-controlled trials on diabetes in a year, and discovered that, in their elegantly-stated one sentence conclusion, "In this sample of registered ongoing RCTs in diabetes, only 18% included patient-important outcomes as primary outcomes."[23]

Researchers often look at "surrogate" or "intervening" vari-ables as their measures, based upon the assumption that previ-ous research has strongly tied these variables to patient-important outcomes. Examples include blood sugar (or glycosylated hemo-globin, hemoglobin A1c) for diabetes, blood pressure, cholester-ol, weight (or body mass index, BMI, a measure of weight-for-height). There is no reason for anyone to care about an asymp-tomatic measure like any of these except to the extent that they are indicators of likely bad patient-important outcomes. However, often the research tying the indicators to bad outcomes is old, or weak, or biased, or all three. Physicians and medical researchers are sometimes so convinced of the association that they do not even question it, as was discussed earlier regarding tight control of blood sugar in diabetes, which can lead to bad outcomes. Thus, we can end up with a plethora of studies measuring surrogate variables that might not be as strongly tied to patient-important outcomes as we believe them to be. Worse, researchers can get carried away and assume that if, say, relatively low blood sugar or cholesterol is good, then even lower is better; this may not be true.

Sometimes the variables being measured are tightly tied to social differences. An example is weight and class. This has important implications for social justice. In popular culture, weight is a major issue. Celebrities are (mostly) thin; when they are not, and look like more of the regular people who are around us, they are seen as unusual. Diet books and "fad" diets abound, as do classes to help us exercise and otherwise lose weight. Body image is a major stressor for adolescents in particular, and health problems like anorexia are all too common. And, yet, an increasing number of Americans are obese, and health problems that are certainly associated with obesity—notably, but not only, Type II diabetes—are rapidly growing.

There is a major class association with weight; as income and class drop, the prevalence of obesity goes up. There is a historical irony to this; in earlier centuries, being heavy was associated with money, that is, the ability of the person to afford all that food, and poor people were starving. Regardless of irony, it is still serious. The abundance of cheap, high-calorie foods in our society means that poor people are no longer denied the opportunity to have lots of calories, but the stressors of poverty that affect all aspects of social life are still there, and obesity becomes one more problem.

There is no question that at some level increased weight results in increased health risk. Body Mass Index (BMI) is the measure usually used because it accounts for weight-for-height. There are established standards for adults: normal is defined as 18.5-25, overweight as 25-30, and obese as greater than 30. Since people can be a *lot* greater than 30, further subdivisions of obesity include "grade 1" (30-35), "grade 2" (35-40) and "grade 3" (>40). Most researchers assume that "normal" is good. They don't become concerned about being underweight until the BMI is less than 18.5 (for reference, a BMI of 18.5 in a 5'8" adult would be 122 lbs.), and consider overweight bad (for that 5'8" person it would be a BMI > 25, or 165 lbs.). Since these seem like pretty low weights for Americans, it would be good to know how strongly these BMIs are tied to patient-important outcomes; maybe they are, and most of us are just various degrees of fat.*

What, in fact, is the value of saying a certain weight (or BMI) is "normal" or "abnormal", beyond the cosmetic? It is only if the "abnormal" can be found to be associated with a higher rate

---

* I am not even sure where the original research that determined these "normal" is from, and I've spent quite a bit of time looking. Each time I think I may have found it, I am disappointed. The CDC website just quotes those as normal. Clinical guidelines on the identification, evaluation, and treatment of overweight and obesity in adults," put out by an expert panel in 1998 ("Clinical guidelines on the identification, evaluation, and treatment of overweight and obesity in adults: executive summary," *Am J Clin Nutr* 68: 899-917, 1998), do not reveal the source of how the "normals" were derived; they are just asserted. Even Wikipedia, while indicating that the measure was devised by a Belgian in the mid-1800s, and was popularized by a 1972 article by Ancel Keys in the *Journal of Chronic Disease* does not tell us how the numbers representing "normal", "overweight" and "obese" were derived. http://en.wikipedia.org/wiki/Body_mass_index

of disease, or more important, poor patient-important outcomes. Indeed, the most recent research using meta-analysis (a method for examining the results of multiple research studies on the same topic) that reviewed 97 studies with over 2.8 million people and encompassing 270,000 deaths has demonstrated that people in the "overweight" group (BMI 25-30) have a *lower* risk for all-cause mortality than those of "normal" weight (18.5-25), and those in the "grade 1" obesity group (BMI 30-35) have the same risk as "normals."[24] In addition, the "hazard ratios" for mortality were greater for the same BMI when heights and weights were self-reported rather than measured (suggesting people under report or underestimate their weight, which would mean their BMIs are actually higher than reported). Why is this a problem? If the medical system pushes people to lose weight, it can not only lead to psychological stress, and be a manifestation of social inequality when weight is unequally distributed among social classes, but lead to health issues as people go on extreme diets. If it turns out that the data are wrong, and the most healthful weight is not what it is purported to be, then there is the possibility of the medical system urging people to a less healthful weight.

This report generated a lot of concern in the obesity-research community because it challenged their core assumptions. This is a little odd, since each of the 97 studies had been out before, but one reason is that people tend to choose which studies to believe. Part of how they do this is the degree to which it confirms their pre-existing beliefs. There was already a sense among many that people at the "low end" of overweight (say with BMI of 26-27) might be as least as healthy (have as low a mortality risk) as those at the low end of "normal." Heymsfield and Cefalu, in an editorial commenting on this study, *Does body mass index adequately convey a patient's mortality risk?*, write:

> *Persons with a BMI between 18.5 and 22 have higher mortality than those with a BMI between 22 and 25. Placing these persons in a single group raises the mortality rate for the normal weight group. The average resulting from combining persons in the lowest mortality category (BMI of 22-25) with those who have greater mortality (BMI of 18.5-22) might explain why the NHLBI category of normal weight has an observed mortality similar to class 1 obesity (BMI of 30-35).*[25]

Of course, if people with a BMI of 18.5-22 have a higher mortality rate than those with a BMI of 25-30, why should we consider 18.5-25 to be normal? The real question is, what are the healthiest ranges to be at? This should be what official recommendations are based on.

The relationship between adiposity (presence of significant amounts of excess fat) and risk for many diseases is well-established; the relationship between adiposity and BMI less well. Variables include amount of muscle mass (not a risk factor but leading to greater weight-for-height), sickness (people whose BMI is low because they have lost weight as a result of disease), and overall body structure. A 2013 op-ed piece in the *New York Times* makes many of these points,[26] but letters generated in response range from those lauding it and saying people (especially children) should be taught to be proud of their bodies, to those arguing it minimizes the health dangers of obesity. What is clear, though, is that the fixation on "ever thinner" that exists in much popular culture has no place in health discussions.

The research strongly suggests that our current standards for "normal" are too low, which means we label people as "over-weight" and "obese" when their BMI may actually be in a health-ful range. This discussion is important as an illustration because in similar areas in which health professionals have likewise adopted uni-dimensional disease markers and aimed to drive them even lower, the result is a tendency toward poorer health outcomes. As I have noted above, related examples include blood sugar (or he-moglobin A1c), blood pressure, and cholesterol. Studies that held everything else equal found benefit in lower values, so experts kept driving down the definitions of "normal" and "desirable" for these tests.

Unfortunately, not everything else in regular people is equal. Pushing the desirable hemoglobin A1c level of people with diabe-tes to 5% instead of 6% led to a lot of morbidity from hypoglyce-mia; lowering cholesterol goals led to toxicities from drugs; low-ering blood pressure goals led to poorer functioning and greater mortality in some populations, especially the elderly. A study by Tinetti, et al.[27], published in *JAMA* found that in a large population of older adults with hypertension, those on medications had a risk of falls, many serious, including those leading to fractures and even to death. This is not to say that high blood pressure should not be treated with drugs, but to point out that discovering a lin-ear relation between treating a condition and decreased morbid-ity *from that condition* misses the fact that the human body is an integral whole, that treating one condition, particularly with drugs, can have adverse effects, and that simply saying "lower blood pressure!," "lower blood sugar!," or "lower cholesterol!," can lead to a shift in the harm/benefit ratio.

It is critical for health professionals to recognize that they are also social service professionals and members of a society whose dominant characteristics and broad policies have a much more profound impact upon health than small numbers variation in BMI, blood pressure, cholesterol, and blood sugar. We need to treat, as well as support and encourage, people at the extremes whose health is at risk, but we shouldn't fall prey to definitions designed to name more people as diseased and needing interventions. This may be good for drug manufacturers and other purveyors of those interventions, but it distracts us from the real business at hand, which is creating a more just, fair, equitable and safe society.

This issue goes far beyond doctors doing things to individual patients that could have been done better. The structural point here is that, because we get into trouble when each indicator is looked at in isolation; we need to be sure that PCPs and other providers consider the whole person. Sure, lower blood sugars, or cholesterol, or blood pressure, or BMI can be good—but would it be good in this person? The answer requires knowledge of that person's larger medical context. And that is something PCPs are good at, but often specialists, focusing on their narrower areas, may miss.

Thus the PCP shortage is more than just a problem of not having enough gatekeepers who can refer people to the right specialist—far from it. The PCP shortage is about whether people get care that is tailored very specifically to who they are. And far from being like a suit, where it's a nice luxury to have one tailored rather than off the rack, tailored health care can mean the difference between life and death.

Beyond having enough PCPs for everyone to have one quarterbacking their health care, and ensuring coordination of care, we need to have an organized health system that rationally looks at benefit for whole people rather than simply a series of individual recommendations for individual diseases by individual specialties and advocacy groups. We need leadership from our medical organizations, and more explicitly from our governmental health agencies, that place each individual disease-focused recommendation into the context of the whole person. Campaigns like *Choosing Wisely* are a good start, but as noted do not distinguish adequately between small "cosmetic" changes and structural changes. Our reimbursement system needs to reward improving health, not "doing things."

As noted previously, a major new initiative of the ACA was the creation of PCORI, designed to not just evaluate new treatments but how they affect people. However, even community-based research has focused largely on the recruitment of research subjects for studies designed by academic researchers, rather than on directly studying issues that would improve the health of the people in those communities. Part of the problem is that it is difficult to get community members to think about what would be in the best interests of their health and that of their communities. They are, after all, not trained to make such an assessment. In addition, particularly in the communities that are the most vulnerable and suffer the greatest health inequities, most people are just focused on getting by, paying the rent, buying food, working multiple low-wage jobs. But another part of the problem is that research at this level is seen as less important and significant, particularly by those who have always focused on new discoveries in the laboratory and who control most of the agencies such as the NIH.

But it is not less important or less significant. No matter how wonderful the discoveries in the lab, no matter how much they might lead to new understanding, new drugs or new treatments, they are only of value if people benefit from them. This requires clinical research in the real world, with actual people. Beyond this, if these interventions are to benefit more than just a chosen few, they have to be studied among diverse populations, including people facing economic, social, psychological and environmental challenges.

Another issue is that, even when we know what an appropriate treatment is, and even when the cost is low enough that people can afford it, we have big gaps in the delivery of these treatments. For example, it has been clearly demonstrated that administration of aspirin is of benefit to people who have had heart attacks. So it should be used. Why, then, are half the Americans who should be on aspirin not taking it? Since it probably isn't cost, what are the reasons? The fact is that it requires research to find out why and to change it. Even though we know what to do, we are not doing it, and we don't know the reason why; finding out how to get this effective treatment to the people who need it is as important as discovering the treatment. Research that looks into why interventions that other research has shown to be effective are not being implemented, known as "fidelity" research, is thus very important.

Finally, effective research on improving people's health needs to involve medical practices, where the people are being seen. There are many Practice-Based Research Networks (PBRNs) around the nation, but they are all challenged by how busy the providers are seeing patients. This is certainly true in practices such as Federally- Qualified Health Centers (FQHCs) that care for poorer populations. And yet, without involving them in research, how can we know what is effective in delivering the "best quality" care, and how can practices at the point of care be changed?

This is not to say that we should not fund basic biomedical research or early clinical trials. Nor is it to say that the current programs from NIH and PCORI and others that fund work in health disparities, inequities, and in population and community health are not good. But they are too little. People working in basic laboratory research, early clinical research, practice-based research, and community health should not be competing with each other. There should be more money for all of it, but especially for those areas that will help to fill the gaps, and learn how to effectively use the information we have to improve people's health. We need "fidelity" research to find out the real reasons why things that we already have good evidence for are not being done, together with community-based participatory research and practice based research.

Research on Disparities/Inequities, in Practices and Communities Need Much Greater Funding

The news is not always good for regular people, and almost never good for poor people. In the U.S. we have the greatest accumulation of wealth and income in the smallest percent of people since the end of the 19th century. CEO salaries have skyrocketed while workers' income has stayed the same, or decreased. (Figure 8.1).[28] This is a problem, but it is made worse by the way in which those with wealth choose to use it, which is largely to further increase their wealth and power. Recent Supreme Court decisions have expanded their ability to contribute to politicians who presumably will continue to work to enhance their wealth. The threat is not just that some people have a lot of wealth, but that a lot of people have nothing, or next to nothing, and that there is strong animus among the powerful toward improving that situation, to enhancing justice in society.

After WWII, President Truman was unsuccessful in passing a national health insurance plan, thanks to both the reactionary opposition of the AMA, and the fact that labor unions chose to demonstrate their effectiveness by negotiating health coverage through collective bargaining rather than seeking political change as the Labour Party successfully did in Britain. In other areas of science, health moved to the forefront. The National Institute of Health (NIH) became the major government institution funding medical research and saw enormous growth in the ensuing decades, including a doubling of the budget from about $15B to about $30B in the decade surrounding the last millennium. This fueled the development of an enormous expansion of medical research in laboratories, primarily in universities and medical schools. In addition, corporate support, mainly from pharmaceutical research companies, further enhanced the growth of these laboratories. There were many successes, of which the most famous is the sequencing of the human genome. Our understanding of human biology and how it might contribute to human health and diseases has been remarkably enhanced. Some of this research has led to true medical breakthroughs, with the creation of new drugs and treatment modalities that have sometimes been of great help to large numbers of people with common diseases, such as diabetes, and sometimes of enormous help to a few with uncommon ones, such as a variety of autoimmune conditions.

However, the focus on laboratory research and new discoveries at the molecular, protein and genetic levels left unfunded areas of research at least as critical, but not seen as "hard science", and thus not generally funded by NIH and drug companies.

Figure 8.1

CEO Pay Compared With Workers' Pay Over 30 Years

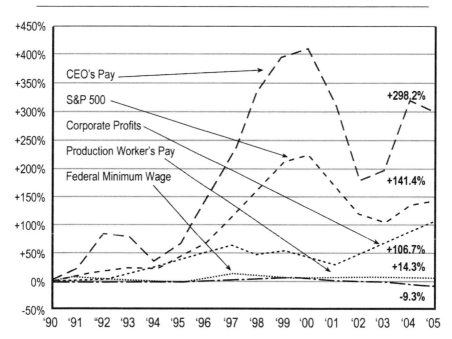

Source: Kavoussi B, CEO Pay grew 127 times faster than worker pay over last 30 years: Study, *Huffington Post,* July 4, 2012. http://www.huffingtonpost.com/2012/05/02/ceo-pay-worker-pay_n_1471685.html

This is a problem. Yes, there are "clinical" research studies, but these are mostly trials of drugs and interventions in populations. We still have only a small number of studies based in communities, looking at health disparities, and trying to discover how to most effectively have a positive influence on the health of people, populations, rather than occasional individuals.

Where will the money come from for this increased research? From policies that are used in every other successful country, and every time the U.S. has been successful: progressive tax policies that take some of our wealth out of the control of private corporations, who use it only to sock away more money, and into the public sector where it can be used to benefit us all.

References

1   Sackett DL, Haynes RB, Evidence base of clinical diagnosis: the architecture of diagnostic research, *Brit M J* 330:1164, 2005.

2   An excellent summary can be found in *Robert Proctor's book Golden Holocaust: Origins of the Cigarette Catastrophe and the Case for Abolition.* University of California Press. 2013.

3   Avorn J, Healing the overwhelmed physician, *New York Times,* June 12, 2013.

4   Ibid # 3.

5   Prasad V, Cifu A, President Bush's unnecessary heart surgery." *Washington Post,* August 9, 2013

6   Marmot M, Sorting through the arguments on breast screening, *JAMA.* 309(24):2553-2554, 2013

7   Kachalia A, Mello MM, Breast cancer screening: conflicting guidelines and mediolegal risk, *JAMA* 309 (24): 2555-2556, 2013.

8   Bleyer A, Welch HG, Effect of three decades of screening mammography on breast-cancer incidence, *N Engl J Med* 2012;367(21):1998-2005. November 22, 2012.

9   Kotz, D. Study links mammograms to overtreatment, *Boston Globe,* November 21, 2012.

10 Woolf SH, Campos-Outcalt D, Severing the link between coverage policy and the US Preventive Services Task Force, *JAMA* 309 (18): 1899-900, May, 2013.

11 Brody H, From an ethics of rationing to an ethics of waste avoidance, *N Engl J Med* 366 (21): 1949-51, May 24, 2012.

12 Ibid # 11

13 Prasad V, Cifu A, Ioannidis JPA, Reversals of established medical practices: evidence to abandon ship, *JAMA* 307(1): 37-8. Jan 4, 2012.

14 Freedman DH, Lies, damned lies, and medical science, *The Atlantic,* November, 2011.

15 *Qaseem A, et al,* Screening Pelvic Examination in Adult Women: A Clinical Practice Guideline From the American College of Physicians, *Annals of Internal Medicine. 161 (1): 67-72. 2014*

16 *New York Times* Editorial Board, The Dispute Over Annual Pelvic Exams http://

www.nytimes.com/2014/07/03/opinion/the-dispute-over-annual-pelvic-exams. html?ref=opinion. July 3, 2014.

17   Choosing Wisely, American Board of Internal Medicine Foundation. http://www. choosingwisely.org/

18   http://www.choosingwisely.org/doctor-patient-lists/american-society-of-clinical-oncology/

19   American Academy of Family Physicians, *Fifteen Things Physicians and Patients Should Question.* http://www.choosingwisely.org/doctor-patient-lists/american-academy-of-family-physicians

20   Allen W, Eggs Benedict, http://www.youtube.com/watch?v=0gtih0PP4kk

21   Murray K, How doctors die, *J Miss State Med Assoc* 54(3):67-9, March 2013

22   Methodology Committee of the Patient Center Outcomes Research Institute, Methodological Standards and Patient-Centeredness in Comparative Effectiveness Research, *JAMA 307 (15): 1636-1640, 2012.*

23   Gandhi GY et al., Patient-important outcomes in registered diabetes trials,*JAMA. 299 (21): 2543-9, June 4, 2008.*

24   Flegal KM, et al. Association of All-cause mortality with overweight and obesity using standard BMI Categories: A systematic review and meta-analysis, *JAMA* 309 (1): 71-82 Jan 2, 2013.

25   Heymsfield SB, Cefalu WT, Does body mass index adequately convey a patient's mortality risk? *JAMA* 309 (1): 87-88, Jan 2, 2013.

26   Campos P, Our absurd fear of fat, *New York Times,* January 3, 2013.

27   Tinetti ME, et al., Antihypertensive medications and serious fall injuries in a nationally representative sample of older adults, *JAMA Intern Med* 174 (4): 588-95. April 1, 2014.

28   Kavoussi B, CEO Pay grew 127 times faster than worker pay over last 30 years: Study, *Huffington Post,* July 4, 2012. http://www.huffingtonpost.com/2012/05/02/ceo-pay-worker-pay_n_1471685.html

Chapter 9

The Role of Profit in U.S. Health Care

The U.S. health care system is not designed to get you the care you need, it is designed to get you the care that someone can make a profit giving you.[1]

—Lee Green, M.D.

Let's be realistic. Employing physicians is not achieving better cost, it's achieving better profit.[2]

—Hospital system Board member to its CFO

"What is its purpose?" is the core question we must ask in creating, assessing, and participating in a health care system. Is it to foster and enhance the health of people, individuals and populations, or to enhance the wealth of those selling it? In a capitalist society, the answer, for most goods and services, is "a balance." We provide a product that helps people—food or cars or clothes—and, if we are good and lucky, make a profit at it. We provide services that people value, and—again if we are good and lucky—make a profit at it. At the ideal (or idealized) extreme, people value something because it is of high quality and meets their needs, pay for it, and the vendor makes an honest margin. At the other extreme, markets are manipulated, goods and services are of low quality, profiteering takes place, and trust is eliminated. We have seen all too much of the latter in recent years because a variety of consumer protections have been either eroded by law (and sometimes by court decisions) or repealed altogether. But this central question remains: should health systems exist for the purpose of creating health for everyone, with reasonable profit made by people who provide necessary and high-quality services at reasonable price, or should they exist to maximize the profit of the providers of goods and services, whether or not people get healthier—or even get quality health care?

Most developed countries, although capitalist, have opted for excluding health from the "unfettered" marketplace because of a shared societal belief that, at least in this area, there needs to be justice; they believe that everyone is entitled to get the health care that they need and have the opportunity to live a healthy life. In the U.S., this is not the case. In part, this is manifested financially; before the Affordable Care Act (ACA) there were tens of millions of people without either health insurance or the money to access health care, and even after it there will still be many millions of uninsured and underinsured. In many places there are powerful forces seeking to increase that number, for example by blocking the expansion of Medicaid.

Health care is a complex business, "business" both in the sense of "a human endeavor" and also as "an organization seeking to make a profit." Over the last several decades we have seen increases in the "for profit" portion of the health care delivery market. Many hospitals have joined the ranks of other parts of the health care industry that have always been predominately for profit, including long-term care facilities, pharmaceutical companies, device makers, home health agencies, and insurance companies.

While "for profit" means that these organizations pay taxes, just because an organization is "not-for- profit" does not mean it behaves significantly differently. Not-for-profits are granted this status because a significant part of their activity is providing a public good, and their income-over-expenses (profit, which we can call "margin" to be less confusing) is not owned by shareholders but is rather intended to be re-invested to further enhance that public good. But not-for-profit hospitals generally follow very similar business practices as their for-profit counterparts. They have to "compete for market share."

While they may have a mission, not-for-profits often cite the mantra "no margin, no mission" as they invest in high-margin "product lines" (generally heart disease, cancer, neurosurgery) to attract more paying customers, rather than spending that money providing their wonderful care for free or at great discount to the poor and uninsured, or in expanding their provision of high-need but low-margin services such as primary care, normal obstetrics, pediatrics, and psychiatry. The salaries paid to the management of not-for-profit hospitals and professional personnel are often as high as those paid by for-profits (who, after all, have to maximize profit to please their shareholders, so want to keep costs, largely salaries, down). Health inequities exist not only because of differences between rural and urban populations, but also because people of different race and ethnicity or of different socioeconomic status do not have the same access to health services. It is not even solely because of the differences in the social determinants of health. It is also because profit has become the *raison d'être* of our health system, and everyone suffers (but the most disadvantaged suffer the most) and no one really even knows what anything costs.

This is clearly an affront to the concepts of health, justice, and equity. Health care business leaders would say that their goal

229

is to make profit, and many critics would agree (casting it as a negative). Greek physician Alex Benos characterized the key relationship between business and health care very well: "Health and health care are not commodities that exist to drive the economy. They are among the social goods that we have an economy in order to be able to achieve."[3] Moreover, businessmen should realize unilateral focus on profit is also a real risk to business. In *How the Mighty Fall*, Jim Collins describes how some of the major companies that he and Jerry Porras had profiled in *Built to Last* later fell because they lost sight of what their core purpose was in pursuit of profit, ironically failing to profit in the final analysis.

George Merck II [of Merck Pharmaceuticals] passionately sought to preserve and improve human life. Paul Galvin [Motorola] obsessed over the idea of continuous renewal through unleashing human creativity. Bill Hewlett and David Packard believed that HP existed to make technical contributions, with profit serving as only a means and measure of achieving that purpose. George Merck II, Paul Galvin, Bill Hewlett and David Packard—they viewed expanding and increasing scale not as the end goal, but as a residual result, an inevitable outcome, of pursuing their core purpose. Later generations forgot this lesson. Indeed, they inverted it.[4]

Is Our Health System Really Free Market?
Has it Ever Been?

The idea that the health industry is somehow, before or after the ACA ("Obamacare") an exemplar of the free market and the success (or not) of private enterprise, is entirely a myth, a facile construct that is used by those making lots of money on the current system to block change. Medicare, a government agency, sets the rates that they will pay for Medicare patients, and private insurers pay multiples of Medicare rates. The entire system is based on this policy; what is profitable is based on what Medicare will pay. For example, it is profitable to provide cancer care because Medicare (and thus other health insurers) pay an enormous amount to administer chemotherapy drugs. Cardiac care, orthopedics and neurosurgical interventions are also very profitable; not so much psychiatry, obstetrics and pediatrics. The doctors who do the profitable things want you to think (and presumably think themselves) that it is because what they do is so hard or that they work so hard; it is in fact a result entirely of regulatory policy. Moreover, a majority of the money spent on "health care" is public funds, not private: Medicare, Medicaid, federal (including military), state and local government employees and retirees, and add in the tax break for employer contributions to health insurance (i.e., taxes forgone because this employee reimbursement is not counted as regular income).

So, if the majority of the money being spent on health care is public money, and the system is already highly government influenced with government policies setting reimbursement rates, the only thing "private" about it is the ownership and profit, both by providers and private insurance companies. Government provides the funds and the private sector makes the money. There is a parallel to our financial services industry: private enterprise is given a license to make money from everyone, and the government finances it. The only difference is that for financial services, the government steps in to bail them out only after they have already taken all our money, while in health services the profit margin is built in from the start. Steven Schroeder of the University of California at San Francisco (quoted in Elisabeth Rosenthal's article *Health Care's Road to Ruin*) notes that "People in fee-for-service are very clever—they stay one step ahead of the formulas to maximize revenue."[5] But, of course, we the people, through our elected representatives and regulators, allow them to do so. And, therefore, the arcane network of incentives and disincentives built into the ACA tries to get reasonable results at reasonable cost—and still ensure insurance companies make lots of profit.

Cui bono? Is healthcare financing about funding providers or caring for patients?

The key question is: what is health care for? Is it about making money for providers and suppliers, or about improving the health of people? This requires an answer, not just once but each time we—governments, policy makers, organizations, professionals, individuals—have to make a decision regarding our health or health system. For example, a few years ago, in New York, there was a conflict between the governor, Andrew Cuomo, and the then-mayor, Michael Bloomberg, about a health insurance company called Emblem moving from non-profit to for-profit status.[6] Cuomo was for it because it could bring as much as $1 billion in tax revenue to state coffers; Bloomberg was concerned because Emblem insured the majority of municipal employees and he feared (with justification, based on previous insurance company conversions from not-for-profit to for-profit) that such a move would drive up the cost of premiums. The governor and mayor were able to "work it out", between them, for the benefit of both the city and state governments, if not necessarily for the people insured by Emblem.

Emblem was, interestingly, created by a merger of Group Health Insurance (GHI) and Health Insurance Plan (HIP) of Greater New York, two early not-for-profit HMOs, or managed care organizations. (They were created so early that it was before either term, HMO or managed care, existed.) In the 1950s and 1960s, these were both consumer cooperatives, established so that by cutting out the for-profit insurance company middleman, people could have more care for the same money, or the same care for less money. It is no wonder that the majority of city employees enrolled.

Over time, rebranded by the Reagan administration with the new name of "HMO", or later managed care, this model became the *de facto* standard for U.S. health care coverage. Conservatives could buy into this vaguely populist or socialist concept because the new HMOs would increasingly be owned by for-profit insurance companies, which they could literally buy into as shareholders. The savings that came from managing care would now accrue to the insurer, not the patient-owner-members. Many of the long-standing HMOs of the early period (e.g., Los Angeles' Ross-Loos) were purchased by insurance companies, but there were a few holdouts that remained consumer cooperatives (e.g., Group Health of Puget Sound as well as the groups that became Emblem). And then, as we remember, came the consumer backlash against HMOs in the late 1990s. People were furious at the restrictions these organizations put on their access to health care. The error, however, was thinking that the cause of the problem was the way that care was organized, such as requirements for only approved therapies, relatively "closed panels" of doctors and hospitals, and capitated payments. In fact, the problem was that they were, and are, mostly owned by for-profit corporations. They increase their profits every time care is denied. This is a very different incentive than when the owners are the patients themselves through a cooperative. Corporatization, not care management, was the cause of their unpopular practices.

As time went on, even the non-profit HMOs and other non-profit groups like the Blue Cross/Blue Shields (BC/BS) have had to act like for-profits in order to compete. In this situation, all advantages have accrued to the insurers, which remain very profitable, rather than to patients, who find many of the same restrictions they bridled at in the past, together with increasing premiums, co-payments, and deductibles. ACA did not really change this, since most of the money being paid for premiums, including the federal subsidies, ends up with insurance companies.

Health industry consulting groups, such as the Advisory Board®, warn hospitals that there will be major cuts to their income resulting from federal budget cuts and programs such as pay-for-performance (P4P) and "value based purchasing" (VBP). (Just to note, VBP, a federal program, is referring to "value" in the economic sense, i.e., cheaper; contrary to what I imagined when I first heard about it, it has nothing to do with "values", such as caring for the sick.) Hospitals worry about whether their historically successful strategy of investing in the highest-profit "product lines", such as heart disease and cancer, will continue to work in the changing reimbursement system. They sense a pressure, as do physicians, to enter into "health system collaborations" in order to maximize efficiency and try to protect profit. There is a certain irony in pressures to re-create the managed care era.

But, because that re-creation is still about how hospitals, doctors, and insurers can make money, not about how we can provide the best health care for the most people, it is essentially a cosmetic change. The current system will be unsustainable if our economy is unable to tolerate ever-increasing portions of our gross domestic product (GDP) going to "health care," squeezing out spending on education, infrastructure improvement, and other social goods, or if people at some point demand that health care dollars are actually spent on health care for people. When the system falters or fails, it will be, as always, the poor who are hurt first and worst, but most of us will suffer.

Throughout 2013 and into 2014, *New York Times* reporter Elisabeth Rosenthal wrote a series of articles on problems with the U.S. healthcare system. One highly-acclaimed piece was called "The $2.7 trillion medical bill: Colonoscopies explain why the U.S. leads the world in health expenditures."[7] She attempts to explain why our costs are much higher than those in other countries but our outcomes are often worse, and large portions of our population are not even covered. Essentially, the reason is greed—on the part of providers (doctors and hospitals), insurers, drug and medical equipment manufacturers to squeeze as much out of us as they can. The reason is that we have a for-profit health care system.

Of course, it is not all colonoscopies. Yes, the average cost for a colonoscopy in the U.S. is $1,155 compared, for example, to $655 in Switzerland. And it is often higher; Rosenthal cites patients who were charged from $6,385 to as much as $19,438. While their insurers negotiated down the price, the final bill for each test was still more than $3,500. Comparisons of U.S. prices with other first-world countries for other common procedures and drugs are likewise striking:

Angiogram: $914 U.S., $35 Canada;

Hip replacement: $40,364 U.S., $7,731 Spain;

MRI: $1,121 U.S., $319 Netherlands;

Lipitor® (atorvastatin, a drug to treat high cholesterol): $124 U.S., $6 New Zealand.[8]

Colonoscopies provide a good example of why we pay so much more for procedures—and it is not because they are of higher quality:

Colonoscopies... are the most expensive screening test that healthy Americans routinely undergo—and often cost more than childbirth or an appendectomy in most other developed countries. Their numbers have increased many fold over the last 15 years, with data from the Centers for Disease Control and Prevention suggesting that more than 10 million people get them each year, adding up to more than $10 billion in annual costs. Largely an office procedure when widespread screening was first recommended, colonoscopies have moved into surgery centers—which were created as a step down from costly hospital care but are now often a lucrative step up from doctors' examining rooms—where they are billed like a quasi operation. They are often prescribed and performed more frequently than medical guidelines recommend. The high price paid for colonoscopies mostly results not from top-notch patient care, according to interviews with health care experts and economists, but from business plans seeking to maximize revenue; haggling between hospitals and insurers that have no relation to the actual costs of performing the procedure; and lobbying, marketing and turf battles among specialists that increase patient fees."[9]

This is a detailed illustration of how, in the U.S., the principle of "maximize profit" determines what health care institutions do. Where "what we do" (our "product") is health care, but we prefer to do it on those with really good insurance. Where we adjust our charges to maximize the difference between what it costs us and what we are paid. Where the rules set by insurers (including government) aimed at regulating costs are seen as challenges to be gamed for maximum profit. Insurers don't negotiate costs with hospitals and doctors for efficiency, but for profit; the more saved, the more their investors get.

Government is different from insurers, certainly. While the government can be motivated to help people by paying for health care, to save taxpayer money by cutting waste, or even denying people health care (to make a political point), it never aims to make a profit. However, as I have pointed out earlier, the government, through Medicare pricing, sets the relative value of different health care services on which the insurance companies base their charges. Thus it is susceptible to pressure from those who do profit by higher charges for procedures.

Moving colonoscopies—and many other procedures—from doctors' offices to "surgi- centers" is a great example of the cost problem. If performing colonoscopies in an office was unsafe, moving them to a surgi-center might be a good idea, but there is little evidence that it was. Moreover, the increased *price* for performing a procedure in such a center far exceeds the increased *cost* of doing it there; the reason for the move is not patient safety, but taking advantage of a loophole to charge more.

Much of the reason for the high cost of health care in the U.S. is the high cost of procedures. It is why procedural specialists, including surgeons who operate and "medical" specialists who do procedures such as colonoscopy, bronchoscopy and dialysis, make so much more than primary care physicians and subspecialists whose practice does not include procedures. This is why decreasing the difference in income potential for proceduralists and primary care doctors would be good for everyone and save money: there would be more people choosing to do primary care and less incentive to do unnecessary procedures. A July 2013 article in *Consumers Report* addressed the high cost of care in the U.S., comparing it specifically to France, which spends 11.6% of its GDP on health care and "...is generally acknowledged as having one of the world's best health care systems." Needless to say, the comparison is not flattering to the U.S., which spends 17.6% of GDP on health care.[10]

The high cost of health care in the U.S. is rarely related to quality, as is illustrated by another article in the *New York Times*, which informs us that, at the time of the article (May 26, 2013), "The most expensive hospital in America is not set amid the swaying palm trees of Beverly Hills or the luxury townhouses of New York's Upper East Side," but Bayonne Medical Center, in Bayonne, NJ, where the average charges are 4.1 times the national average and much higher than what Medicare will pay. For some services it is much higher:

Bayonne Medical typically charged $99,689 for treating each case of chronic lung disease, 5.5 times as much as other hospitals and 17.5 times as much as Medicare paid in reimbursement. The hospital also charged on average of $120,040 to treat transient ischemia, a type of small stroke that has no lasting effect. That was 5.6 times the national average and 23.6 times what Medicare paid.[11]

How can they get away with this? Who will pay them so much? After all, if I can buy a Chevrolet for $25,000 at one dealer in town, why would I pay $75,000 for the same car somewhere else? The answer is: health care is different. For one thing, speed and convenience can be important; you might be sick when you have to find a hospital to care for you, and you might live in Bayonne.

Of course, Medicare will only pay what Medicare pays. But if you have most types of commercial insurance (or if you are uninsured), it is another story. To guard against excessively inflated charges, most insurers have contracts with providers (hospitals, doctors, etc.) that determine how much insurers will pay for a procedure or treatment of a disease. This saves the insurer money. In addition, in order to encourage you to go somewhere where they have negotiated these lower rates, so-called "in-plan" hospitals, if you go "out of plan", your insurer will pay a lower percent of the cost—and you will pay more. Thus we have a seeming paradox: insurance companies aim to cut costs by restricting care and capping prices, in order to preserve profit for their investors, while hospitals and other for profit providers seek to provide more care, even unneeded care, at higher prices for exactly the same reasons—to preserve profits for their investors. In a sense, the system is designed as a war between providers and insurers, each trying to satisfy their investors to the maximum extent possible. Lost in the war between these two sides are patients, who just want appropriate care so they can get the best health outcome possible. In this system, it's no wonder that health outcomes suffer.

Recalling Batalden's Law, this is the heart of the design of the system. The ideology of the market is that it offers efficiency and reduced prices through competition. That's often true when you have producers competing to deliver great deals to consumers—consumers can get increasingly great deals. But when both sides have investors, and when competition is blunted or eliminated (because, contrary to the theories of some health economists, consumers can't really comparison shop for health care), then it's a competition for satisfying investors, by raising prices and lowering costs. Insurance companies raise premium prices and lower their costs of medical care. Hospitals raise care prices for the same reason: earn profit for investors.

And it is precisely this effort to control costs that many for-profit hospitals (like Bayonne) have used to generate greater income. They have gone "out of plan" for all health plans. This means that when you show up in their ER, or are admitted to the hospital, you have a higher co-pay and co-insurance charge, and the insurer pays them more money. This is why the insurer doesn't want you to go there, and you might not want to go there either (once you know this). Except, of course, you're sick, and you live in Bayonne, and it is the closest ER, so you are trapped. Winner: Bayonne Medical Center.

This strategy has, at its extreme, the almost bizarre outcomes reported by Elisabeth Rosenthal in the *New York Times*. After surgery, a man recieved a surprise $117,000 medical bill from a doctor he didn't know. The "in-plan" surgeon received $6,200 for his hip replacement, but the assistant surgeon, who was out-of-plan, received, yes, $117,000![12]

It is not just that there are a few hospitals that are, like Bayonne, taking maximum advantage of this system to beat the "competition" of the insurance companies (forget the patient!). The Center for Medicare and Medicaid Services (CMS) issued a report revealing dramatic differences in the prices charged for medical services between hospitals, not only between regions but also within the same city.[13] This report provided many examples cited by a variety of news outlets. From the *New York Times:*

A hospital in Livingston, N.J., charged $70,712 on average to implant a pacemaker, while a hospital in nearby Rahway, N.J., charged $101,945...In Saint Augustine, Fla., one hospital typically billed nearly $40,000 to remove a gallbladder using minimally invasive surgery, while one in Orange Park, Fla., charged $91,000. ...In one hospital in Dallas, the average bill for treating simple pneumonia was $14,610, while another there charged over $38,000.[14]

Bloomberg News noted that treatment of psychoses "showed the greatest price discrepancies, with the most expensive hospital charging $144,523, more than 52 times its cheapest peer," and the "most common procedure in the data, treatment of simple pneumonia and lung inflammation with complications, had prices ranging from $5,093 to as much as $124,051."[15]

These examples are similar to the wide gaps in prices above between U.S. costs and costs in other countries discussed in Chapter 2—except these are gaps between hospitals inside the U.S.. But, of course, this information is no surprise to hospitals and physicians. Investigative journalists have reported on these issues for many years, including Atul Gawande in his article "The Cost Conundrum" in *The New Yorker* and Steven Brill's "Bitter Pill: Why Medical Bills are Killing Us," in *Time.*[17] While each hospital has a "charge master" that lists "list prices" for any number of procedures and equipment (and which, as noted above, vary wildly), Medicare does not pay those prices or anything close to them; it sets its own payment schedule for these procedures, which does not vary much between hospitals. However, as Gawande makes clear, there is a second problem arising from the fact that some hospitals seem to do (and bill Medicare for) a far larger number of procedures than are done by other hospitals caring for similar populations. Because the health status and mortality rate is not greater for people served by those hospitals doing fewer procedures, it is unlikely that the problem is that those hospitals are not doing enough. The more likely explanation is that those doing more are doing some of them unnecessarily.

So, if Medicare pays a set amount, why do hospitals have such high charges and why do they vary so wildly? It is because there are a few insurers whose payments are tied to charges rather than Medicare rates, but also because, of course, some people are not insured. Some of the variation is in "fixed costs", the expenses that hospitals have that are not for the individual patient (staff, building maintenance, equipment, etc.) that are loaded into these charges, as is greater or less profit. The Health and Human Services (HHS) secretary at the time, Kathleen Sebelius, quoted by Reuters, said that:

> When consumers easily compare the prices of goods and services, (providers) have strong incentives to keep those prices low. But even basic information about health premiums and hospital charges has long been hidden from consumers. These rates can vary dramatically in ways that can't be easily explained.[18]

In addition to not having this information easily available, price information is of value mostly in a competitive market; in a monopoly, price matters less. You can possibly choose a different airline if you don't like the service on one, but if you don't like the way the airport in your city works, you're out of luck. It is not clear that posting the prices, or having smaller differences, would be of much help to most consumers; maybe you're sick, and you live in Bayonne.

Like CMS, most large health insurers do not pay listed charges; although they pay more than Medicare or Medicaid, their payments to hospitals are usually a multiple of Medicare charges (e.g., they might pay 150% of Medicare's charges). Of course, the group of people who do get billed for the list price are those people with no insurance at all. The difference between a charge of $24,874 from Truman Medical Center Lakewood and $66,268 from the University of Kansas Hospital for hip replacement surgery is irrelevant to Medicare and large insurers, who pay what they are going to pay. But it is huge to an uninsured person. And while it may even be largely theoretical to them because they are very unlikely to be able to pay those charges, it can, and frequently does, absorb their life savings, ruin their credit, and throw them into bankruptcy. Also there are "middle class" uninsured families who might be able to pay off $24,874 over several years, but for whom $66,268 is more than they could pay in a lifetime.

The structure of medical care pricing is not only opaque, but according to H. Gilbert Welch, a professor of medicine at the Dartmouth Institute for Health Policy and Clinical Practice, it is outrageous. In a *New York Times* Op-Ed, Welch states that he is:

...not talking about a violation of federal or state statutes, like Medicare or Medicaid fraud, although crime in that sense definitely exists. I'm talking instead about the violation of an ethical standard, of the very 'calling' of medicine.[19]

The problem is that the ethical standard that Welch feels is being violated is not part of the system. Rather, the system is designed to avoid these ethical standards; *we have the standards we designed for.* Welch carefully describes both the incredible increase in prices for medical care and the excess use of the procedures that cost the most. He adds that the prices are only partially felt by the end-user (people) because Medicare, Medicaid and commercial insurers pay far lower amounts than the posted prices. However, he adds that the portion paid by people (co-pays, co-insurance, deductibles) is going up, and of course the uninsured are charged full price. "They are largely young and employed (albeit poorly) and have little education," he writes, although in fact many are older, and unemployed (remember Medicaid insures only poor people, but far from all poor people).

Welch's description of the ridiculous prices for medical supplies ($108 for a $5 tube of ointment, etc.) is reminiscent of the $100 hammers bought by the Defense Department several decades ago, except there is a huge difference: because the Defense Department's budget is spread out across hundreds of millions of tax payers, it can survive the outrageous waste. And it can battle it with hired guns who take suppliers to court. But an individual faces a much bigger hardship financially and can't fight back. Welch also discusses the impact of the less well-known increase in charges resulting solely from the purchase of physician practices by hospitals. Hospitals can charge the higher fees that Medicare allows them to, called facility fees. This, legally, resulted in the amount paid by Medicare for an electrocardiogram to increase from $200 to $471, and for a colonoscopy from $2,000 to $8,000, in one year for the same procedure in the same location.

There is a significant irony here: Hospitals are expensive places because they do a lot of expensive things with high tech equipment, and they need to be reimbursed for the infrastructure required to make those things possible. But grouping physician practices together in a hospital saves money and should result in savings passed along to the consumer. Consider: which is more expensive in terms of overhead and infrastructure: 50 doctors located in one building or 50 physician practices located in 50 different buildings? The irony is that, under the guise that it is more expensive to have something done in a hospital, hospitals can charge added facilities fees for having centralized practices and cutting costs!

Welch says that "The word 'crime' is awfully strong. Many prefer to call all this a problem of perverse incentives: good people, working in a bad system." But it is pretty clear that he has not convinced himself, not to mention me. I know the pressures that physicians and hospitals are under to make more money. After all, hospitals are run by businessmen, and buying up all those physician practices and having to pay the doctors does not come cheap, especially when insurers, particularly Medicare, are focusing on saving money by reducing their reimbursements. What appears— correctly—to be an effort to maximize charges, thus increasing the cost to the individual, insurer, and government—is seen by hospitals as a core strategy of survival to make money in a challenging and competitive environment. But a key premise of this book is that we have a system designed to get the results that it gets, and this includes condoning such practices as legal. The question is, do we want a system that condones such immoral behavior, or one that explicitly makes it illegal?

Of course, there is also clear fraud, most often identified in medical suppliers. Federal hearings were held on one such case by Sen. Claire McCaskill of Missouri. They were instigated by communication from a St. Louis physician who informed the Senator that she was receiving requests from medical device sellers for approval of medical equipment that she hadn't ordered, and that it turned out her patients hadn't requested. The idea was that the government would pay for it, so it was "free" to the doctor and patient. At the hearing Senator McCaskill said "Most Americans have seen ads on TV or received calls or letters promising medical equipment 'at little or no cost to you,' ...[but] there is always a cost to you, because it is paid for by federal tax dollars." Patients of both the original doctor and others testified that they often receive several calls per day from device retailers. Investigations of two companies that had faxed unsolicited requests to that physician discovered, respectively, a 68% and 92% "error rate", a euphemism for what may well be fraud.[20]

Sen. McCaskill's committee discovered many cases where patients did not want the equipment that their physicians were asked to approve. There are many others cases in which the patient is convinced that it would be good to have, say, a scooter that they don't have to pay for—even when the doctor thinks it is not necessary or might even be harmful (for example, when a person who doesn't exercise because of their weight gets a scooter and is even less active and thus gains more weight). Fraud is fraud, should be investigated, and it exists; it is indeed one of the benefits for having government financing of health care.

For hospital charges, which are not fraud, however, the solution is to have a single-payer system that, possibly with regional differences based on the cost of labor and other variables, pays a fixed amount for services, as does Medicare. Medicare indeed is not perfect, but a little rationality would go a long way. Medicare may currently pay too little, requiring private insurers to subsidize that care; certainly the law should prevent billing of the uninsured above what Medicare would pay.

Dr. Welch says that "Medical care is intended to help people, not enrich providers." This is reminiscent of another quotation from Rudolph Virchow, the Father of Social Medicine (see Chapter 1): "Medical education does not exist to provide students with a way to make a living, but to ensure the health of the community . . . If medicine is really to accomplish its great task, it must intervene in political and social life."[21]

The problem is that there is an enormous industry built around medical care and providers (doctors, hospitals and owners of various for-profit facilities, the pharmaceutical and device industries, and insurance companies) who are indeed getting very rich. And many of them are running scared that their riches will decrease. If we want a medical care system that is primarily intended to help people rather than enrich providers, we need a major change in the way that it is paid for. We need to devise a system that encourages the provision of high-quality, appropriate care to everyone who needs it, and does not provide unnecessary or potentially harmful care to anyone. We need a system that is not so complicated that it encourages workarounds to cherry-pick profitable patients or perform more profitable procedures. The profit-making competitive marketplace may work for many goods and services, but has no place in our health care.

In the article cited previously, Bavley quotes Robert Zirkelbach, vice president of America's Health Insurance Plans, the industry's trade association. 'When a hospital buys a practice, its rates will increase in the following year's contract. Increases of 20, 30 or 40 percent are not uncommon. It's not 3 or 4 percent, that is for sure.'[22]

To be clear, this is a health insurance executive worried about hospitals jacking up the costs of care—and no wonder; increased health care costs mean either the insurance companies must charge those who buy the premiums more, or do with less profit, or both. That's bad for business (and horrifying for anyone who lacks a great insurance plan). But this is how the system "works": hospitals raise prices (by moves like taking PCPs in-house) so they can preserve profits for their investors, or so they can compete with other hospitals and survive, or both. Insurance companies work to deny care or restrict it to preserve profits or survive, or both. And patients are the biggest losers. Bavley illustrates this with examples of people who were referred internally (within the hospital system) and had delayed diagnosis, or were discouraged from going to another facility for a second opinion. Sometimes it is fine to see doctors within the system, and certainly this can be, and is, encouraged. But discouraging people from seeking outside referrals can also be hazardous to their health.

Physicians and the Cost of Care

The outrage that Dr. Welch expresses in his *New York Times* piece is particularly addressed to physicians, who he believes have a "calling", whose responsibility is to help people.[23] While there are many people and companies out there who are making, or seeking to make, a profit on delivering health care, physicians are also not free from blame for its high cost. Yes, physicians are increasingly employed by health systems and having their practices prescribed by those systems. But to a large extent, physicians control many of the expenditures, and thus the cost of care, because they are the ones who order the tests, prescribe the medicines, use the devices, refer to each other, and advise their patients regarding the most appropriate treatment. To the extent that physicians (and other providers who have this power) exert it wisely, judiciously, and appropriately, the cost of care might begin to be controlled. Yes, there will still be tensions between cost and benefit, between benefit to a single person and benefit to the whole population, between what the goals of care are, and the degree to which physician choices are limited. But cost consciousness among physicians would go a long way. However, the cost consciousness has to compete with the incentive for making money, and it is unlikely that we will succeed in getting physicians to alter their behavior in a way that earns them less. Note that one of the more publicized recommendations from the *Choosing Wisely* campaign, sponsored by the American Board of Internal Medicine Foundation and discussed in Chapter 8, is not to image low back pain for 6 weeks. This recommendation comes from the American Academy of Family Physicians, but is not mentioned by the American College of Radiology or the American Academy of Orthopedic Surgeons. Self-interest, especially financial, is a powerful motivator. So we need an external limit placed, and that limit, rather than being punitive, should be paying for care that is evidence based—for everyone who needs it—and not paying for care that is ineffective, for anyone.

There is evidence that physicians do not see themselves at fault. A random survey of U.S. physicians published in *JAMA* revealed that most did not believe that physicians had any major responsibility for controlling health care costs; it was "the other guys":

Most believed that trial lawyers (60%), health insurance companies (59%), hospitals and health systems (56%), pharmaceutical and device manufacturers (56%), and patients (52%) have a "major responsibility" for reducing health care costs, whereas only 36% reported that practicing physicians have "major responsibility." [24]

The biggest flaw of the survey is that it does not offer a choice of an alternate system. It does not recognize that our present system is designed to make profit rather than to produce health. A two-thirds majority of doctors may think that they are doing all they can already, within the limits of their ethical responsibilities to their patients. But their responses to other questions in the survey cast doubt as to whether they actually are doing all they can, or even think that they are. While "More than 90% of physicians expressed some or strong enthusiasm for improving conditions for evidence-based decisions, including 'expanding access to quality and safety data,' 'promoting head-to-head trials of competing treatments,' and 'limiting corporate influence on physician behavior,'" only 51% were strongly enthusiastic with another 38% "somewhat enthusiastic", about "limiting access to expensive treatments with little net benefit." While it is good that 89% of doctors are somewhat in favor of limiting access to treatment that is of limited benefit (thus the article's contention that it was "relatively strong support"), it is still of concern that nearly half of all doctors are less than strongly enthusiastic about their role in containing health care costs.

When it comes to physician reimbursement, it is unsurprising that doctors are very chary of any new models, since most have been doing pretty well with the old ones. Thus, only 7% supported elimination of "fee-for-service" (FFS), in which doctors get paid for what they do, as opposed to capitation, where they get a fixed amount for caring for their patient. In the capitation system of payment, there is zero incentive to do unnecessary procedures, while under FFS, doctors get paid more for doing more. In the current FFS system, they get paid whether what they do is necessary or not, and paid a *lot* more for doing procedures, rather than getting a global fee for providing care. It is also not surprising that those physicians who were paid salary only or salary-plus-bonus were more than three times as likely to support the elimination of FFS. Self-interest is indeed a powerful motivator, but it is not an insurmountable hurdle. It is why we need systems that encourage doctors to do the right thing rather than the profitable thing by eliminating the incentives to do more.

The authors of an accompanying editorial, apparently searching for some good news, note that:

...51% strongly disagreed that the cost of a test or medication is only important if the patient has to 'pay for out of pocket...'." How much hope does it give you that half of doctors do not strongly disagree that cost of medication is only an issue if it is coming directly out of a patient's pocket? I imagine it is very reassuring to pharmaceutical

companies. Doctors can, and should, be advocates for the interests of their patients, including their patients' ability to pay for medication.[25]

Physicians often rail at "government intrusion" on the physician-patient relationship, and are fond of challenging the medical credentials of administrators who make rules restricting practice. Sometimes those complaints are justifiable, as for example when politicians make rules that limit the access of women to core health care services such as contraception. At other times, when guidelines are put in place to restrict the use of unproven, non-beneficial, and potentially dangerous care, it is much less justified. It is very difficult to make decisions about what is the best treatment even when just considering risk/benefit to the individual, not to mention the harder-to-measure (and more controversial) work of balancing benefit to the individual with benefit to the whole society. It is much easier for someone else to make those decisions, allowing you to be free to criticize them and tell your patients "it's not my fault." But you cannot have it both ways. If it requires regulation and guidelines to ensure inappropriate care is not provided (for example, giving narcotics for head colds), this should not be protested by doctors. While any individual physician might always do the right thing, it is absurd to expect that the right thing will always be done by every individual physician, especially in circumstances where it might be in their financial interest to do otherwise.

Yes, if physicians want to continue to have significant autonomy in the decisions that they make, they need to take on responsibility for the impact. Saying "I just made this decision because it was best for my patient and I can't be responsible for overall health costs" is a little like saying that the candy bar wrapper you just chucked out the window of your car isn't responsible for the garbage all over our roads. More important, and concerning, is the finding that they demonstrate little sense of responsibility for choosing the *right* treatment, rather than the newest or most expensive, even for the individual. There will need to be systemic solutions, guidelines and regulations. This becomes even more true as, increasingly, physicians are becoming employed by hospitals and health systems, a circumstance that is likely to further put pressure on them to order diagnostic tests and treatments that are profitable for their institution.

Alan Bavley of the *Kansas City Star* reported in early 2014 that:

> *Since 2000, the number of doctors on hospital payrolls nationwide has risen by one-third, according to the American Hospital Association. In the Kansas City area, fully 55 percent of physicians are now employed by hospitals, Blue Cross and Blue Shield of Kansas City estimates. That includes virtually all cardiologists and most cancer specialists.* [26]

These changes were not limited to the KC area; Bavley cites both national data and those from disparate regions such as Spartanburg, SC and Phoenix, AZ. Part of the reason, the "financial model", is that such "integrated" practices generate internal referrals, keeping patients within the system, as well as generating lucrative procedures. Physicians get a piece of the action; they get guaranteed salaries paid in part by the hospital or health system that is getting downstream revenue for their referrals. And it makes these hospitals and health systems a lot of money, because of the previously mentioned facility fees, but also through in-creasing "consolidation" of the market, with hospitals becoming oligopolies. This is documented in a June 2014 *New York Times* article "Hospital Charges Surge for Common Ailments, Data Show," by Julie Creswell, Sheri Fink and Sarah Cohen.[27] A follow up *New York Times* editorial discussed the risks of hospital merg-ers as illustrated by the consolidation of two big hospitals in Bos-ton, Massachusetts General Hospital and Brigham and Women's Hospital, which has led to higher charges.[28]

The ethics of the physician's role was addressed by Drs. Da-vid B. Reuben and Christine K. Cassel in a *JAMA* article "Physi-cian stewardship of health care in an era of finite resources." They focus not on how much physicians earn (salary or profit), but how they choose to spend health care dollars, because:

> *Health care costs are directly related to decisions made in clinical practice."* [They go on to say that]: *"These deci-sions are difficult to influence because they are made in the context of individuals who are often sick and vulnerable, with little understanding of the potential benefits and risks of diagnostic and therapeutic options. Patients seek help from physicians and physicians chose careers to provide this help, or at least the hope of it. Because of this relation-ship, it is futile to expect that changing physicians' behav-ior through evidence and shared decision making alone will solve the problem of high health care costs. Alternative ap-proaches will be necessary.[29]*

Cassel, president of the National Quality Forum who in the past was the President and CEO of the American Board of Inter-nal Medicine (ABIM, the organization that certifies internists), is both a geriatrician and a medical ethicist. She has long argued that the use of resources ordered by an individual physician for an individual patient should not be based on considerations other than the benefit and risk for that patient, since the physician and patient have no control over what money "saved" might be used for. (That is, my patient and I cannot decide to forego expensive interventions and instead use the money for housing the homeless or feeding the hungry; all we can decide is whether to do those interventions or not.) Savings have to be looked at on a more global level, with a shared understanding of what those "saved" dollars will be used for, and other than publicly financed care (Medicare, Medicaid, military, VA, etc.) this is virtually impossible in our current system.

Reuben and Cassel provide a taxonomy of physician stewardship, examining the various levels at which it can occur beyond that of individual patient decisions. These include the "highest" level, of national and state policy where spending decisions (initially, one presumes, via Medicare and Medicaid) should be based on evidence of benefit and consistency with national policy objectives (such as, I imagine, *Healthy People 2020*).[30] The second level is that of payers (insurers) who would choose to pay for interventions that are shown to be beneficial (and presumably cost effective) rather than those that are ineffective or marginal. They suggest that rather than charging high deductibles and co-pays for services that are known to be beneficial and cost-effective, insurers simply do not pay for those that are not. The suggestions that they make seem reasonable, and are, but they miss the most important point. No one should pay for procedures that do not work, while health insurance should pay for medically necessary care which they frequently do not (e.g., hearing aids). The systemic flaw once again, is that the system is designed to make profit, not to improve health; anything that an insurance company saves by not paying for a procedure goes to the insurance company, not to providing health care for more people. This would, of course, be solved by a single-payer national health insurance program.

The third level that Reuben and Cassel address is the practice level, where groups of physicians can use evidence to guide their group decision-making and decrease inappropriate variation in physician practice. An example of this would be the use of a limited drug formulary emphasizing generic medications (this could also occur at the insurer level). Finally, there is the individual patient level; while making cost-effective decisions at this level can be more complex, it can certainly be done. A sick person cannot be asked to decide upon the choice of having, or not having, a medical intervention that they can scarcely understand so that saved dollars may possibly benefit some unnamed person. What will actually happen is that saved dollars will provide more money to the insurance company. This is quite a different thing from the good practice of educating people about the impact of their health decisions, especially before they become critically ill. Advance directives, such as living wills and durable powers of attorney for health care (DPOAs), are one method; these, however, are about making wise decisions to benefit them, not about benefiting others except for cases when, for example, they may function as an organ donor.

What is clearly unethical and unacceptable is for physicians to encourage patients, sick or well, to undergo a diagnostic or therapeutic intervention because the physician stands to gain financially from doing it. Unfortunately, this happens. Sometimes it is done consciously, but often it is because the physician who does the procedure truly believes it is of benefit. For a physician whose income depends upon doing the procedure to not believe it would be beneficial would in fact be cognitive dissonance.

Although there are large numbers of procedures that are questionable for anyone, there are far more that are of benefit to some people but not to others. Physicians must be both able to distinguish between these people and present recommendations honestly and free of financial bias. This would make a big difference in reducing the overall cost of health care, but it is extremely unlikely that decisions free from financial bias could ever occur. Even if they could, the idea of ensuring that millions of decisions a day are made on this basis is absurd. Rather, it makes much more sense to reduce financial bias by legislation or clinical practice guidelines. This means having a different system, since the one we have gets the results that it gets. The fact that there are still many physician-owned for-profit hospital and "surgicenters," in which the doctors benefit financially from more procedures, not only as the providers but as owners of the facility, means that the entire way our system is structured is to encourage such behavior.

The greed of human beings is not going to be wished away, whether they are physicians or lay corporate executives; whether of for-profit or not-for-profit companies. The taxonomy of Reuben and Cassel is useful for thinking about these issues, but only comprehensive, thoughtful and balanced regulation that can be sufficient impetus to make these changes happen.

Another way of thinking about this problem is offered by Christopher Moriates and colleagues, in a *Viewpoint* piece in *JAMA* titled "First, Do No Financial Harm." It argues that in this context physicians have four responsibilities. The first two are innovative and good ideas:

1. *Screen for financial harm, i.e., what will it cost this person out of pocket and can they afford it?;*

2. *Adopt a universal approach, i.e., do with everyone. As with HIV screening, or asking about risk behaviors, don't assume you can "tell" who is at risk; doing it with everyone means those you ask are not being "singled out", and you don't miss addressing the issue with people who don't "look like" they'd have a problem.*

The last two responsibilities are less innovative but equally important, and address what I have discussed above:

3. *Understand financial ramifications and value of recommendations.*

4. *Optimize care plans for individual patients.[31]*

Actually, if one looks at past health reforms, physicians as a group have never been in the lead. The American Medical Association (AMA) opposed and was instrumental in defeating President Truman's national health insurance proposal and strongly opposed Medicare in 1965. Change *is* hard, and it is particularly hard when there is a good chance that change will not be beneficial for your pocketbook (of course, as it turns out, the AMA was wrong about Medicare even by this criterion).

We may be cautiously optimistic that a number of physician polls suggest that a majority of physicians favor a single-payer system. In any case, change is necessary. In order to reduce costs and re-engineer the system, and to ensure that money is not wasted, and that quality of care is high, people need to trust in their providers. The ethical principle of *justice*—that everyone with the same conditions has access to the same diagnostic and treatment options—must be adhered to.

"The Thousand Dollar Pap Smear": Bundling Tests and Blaming the Victim

Much of the increase in cost in medical care is an insidious kind of cost "creep" that results from new tests that might be more effective but, like new drugs that might be more effective, carry very much higher price tags. Unlike the drugs, the new tests are often simply put in place by laboratories to replace previous tests without physicians even having a choice in ordering them. In addition, they are frequently "bundled" together with other tests, so if you want test "A" you also get test "B" (or, in fact, tests "B" through "K," or sometimes "ZZ") which may or may not be helpful, but which add significant cost. The whole package may be a bargain compared to getting each test individually, but if you only needed 1, 2 or 3, getting all 20 can cost a lot more.

These factors, "creep" and "bundling", are well illustrated by Cheryl Bettigole in a *NEJM* piece called "The Thousand Dollar Pap Smear."[32] She begins by describing a call from one of her patients, who complained she had been charged over $600 for her Pap smear, shocking both of them. She goes on to describe the beneficial role that Pap smears have had, at least in developed countries. Indeed, this test remains the best example we have of an effective screening test for any cancer. It is also—or should be—very cost-effective based on previous studies, but these studies assumed a $20-$30 cost for the test. So how did it get to be so expensive? Was the price increase really necessary? A portion of the increased cost comes from the use of a more effective and more expensive method of preserving and analyzing the specimen (i.e., "creep"), but most of it comes from including a bunch of other tests ("bundling"). These include tests for human papilloma virus (HPV), recommended only for some women and at intervals less frequently than routine Paps, and tests for sexually-transmitted infections (STIs) which may or may not be indicated based on the patient's history and symptoms but are quite different from cervical cancer screening. In fact, the physician *could* just order the specific tests that she wants, but the laboratory, which makes money on this, "bundles" them into an easy-to-order "panel" of tests (almost never accompanied by the price), and busy clinicians check them off.

Beyond the initial cost of ordering more tests than planned, this also creates the situation where a test, planned or unplanned, shows an unanticipated—and frequently unimportant—abnormality that requires more tests to follow up. This is common not only for Pap smears but for many other lab tests, and contributes to the increased cost of health care for society, insurers, and individuals. Dr. Bettigole points out the role of the provider in contributing to this unnecessary cost by not ordering tests more carefully. She writes:

When I was in training, our attendings would ask a standard quiz question: 'What is the biggest driver of health care costs in the hospital?' Answer: the physician's pen. A mouse or a keyboard, rather than a pen, now drives the spending, but we physicians and our staff are responsible for ordering these unnecessary tests and hence responsible for the huge bills our patients are receiving. [33]

Certainly this is largely correct, and providers should all be careful to order tests (and treatments) cost-effectively and teach our students the same. But this is not the sole answer; it should not require a heroic effort on the part of a provider to know what each test costs, alone or in combination with others. The systems that we have should encourage this sort of test ordering. It should be more difficult, not easier, to do things that are not cost effective. Electronic health records (EHRs) could be helping by providing us with clear comparisons of ordering options and putting prices on each, rather than simply making it easier to click on the most costly choice, but in fact they often compound the problem.

There is a parallel here to victim blaming. We should encourage our patients (and ourselves) to adopt healthful behaviors—a good idea, but not the answer for improving the health of a society so heavily geared to encouraging poor behaviors such as drinking alcohol, smoking tobacco, guns, overeating and eating empty calories, etc. The concept that the "problem" is individuals' bad behaviors often appears to be ubiquitous. Such an attitude is not only victim blaming but is an impractical approach to problem solving. In industry, a strategy called "six-sigma" has been widely adopted; its goal is to make bad outcomes resulting from individual error occur with a frequency approaching zero. Often the example used is aviation, eliminating airplane crashes. It works because systems are put into place that make things work rather than saying to each pilot "Be careful! Remember to push the joystick in the right direction!" Of course, even in aviation, things could be improved; pilots still have the ability to turn off the plane's tracking device. But the options to do unsafe or unwise things remain much greater in medicine.

The Affordable Care Act (ACA) encourages the creation

of "Accountable Care Organizations" (ACOs), which would be responsible (at least hopefully, in the best of scenarios) for the health of a population. At a minimum, ACOs would decrease the degree to which the delivery of health care is a series of episodic events paid for individually, rather taking on a global responsibility including inpatient, outpatient, and long-term care. This would, in theory, change the usual patient experience from seeing one (or many) doctors or having one (or many) ER visits, each charged and paid separately, culminating in a hospitalization, and then discharge to one (or many) doctors, or a long-term care facility (paid separately), and failure of care resulting in readmission to the hospital (paid again). The idea is that all levels would be coordinated to provide the best care at the most appropriate level (inpatient, outpatient, long-term, home based). In some settings, particularly for fully-integrated plans such as Kaiser where the providers of care are also the insurers, this works relatively well.

However, as the second article in Bavley's series makes clear,[34] there is often a great cost to those who are paying, the patient and their insurer (including Medicare and Medicaid). This is because, as discussed earlier in the work of Elisabeth Rosenthal of the *New York Times,* Medicare (and, private insurers following Medicare's lead) pays an additional fee (the "facility fee") for services, and especially procedures, done in a hospital outpatient facility beyond what they would pay for it to be done in a doctor's office.

Why should this be? The original intent, as is often the case, was good, to both save money and improve care, by having many procedures done in outpatient rather than inpatient settings, where the cost would be even higher. And, as is also so often the case, the providers realized that this system could be gamed as well. The physician fee for a visit or procedure done in an office is greater than that done in a hospital clinic, but is expected to include all the overhead. In a hospital-based clinic there is a somewhat lower doctor's fee, but there is also a facility fee that, together with the doctor's fee, is much higher in total than the office-based reimbursement; indeed, the facility fee can be far higher than the physician fee. Hospitals are encouraged to move procedures from inpatient to outpatient, saving money. However, often procedures that were previously done in a doctor's office, are moved to a hospital outpatient setting, thus increasing the cost.

In fact, to qualify for this just means that the office has to be owned by the hospital or health system; it doesn't have to be on the hospital campus and can even be in the same office it was previously. Through this change in ownership, the hospital makes money, and can share some of that with the physician, allowing the physician to make much more money without the overhead and risk. *Voilà*! Physicians are incentivized to become employed by hospitals.

Medicare is, sadly, responsible for much of this situation, as illustrated by the following: seeking to reduce costs for unnecessary admissions, Medicare has empowered bounty hunters (called "RACs") to go after Medicare "fraud" by reviewing admissions to hospitals for patients who could have been cared for in the hospital on "observation" status, which will save Medicare money. Hospitals are thus very careful to only officially "admit" people who meet very strict criteria. However, because "observation" status is officially "outpatient", while Medicare saves money the patient pays more out of pocket, because it is now covered under Medicare Part B, not the Part A that covers hospitalization. This is complicated, but what it comes down to is what is financially good for Medicare is financially bad for the patient. Is this what we want?

I hope not. The real problem is that we do not have a straight-forward system to deliver the highest-quality, necessary, health care to all people but a mess of conflicting incentives. Yes, some of the fault belongs to Medicare, and some of the fault belongs to providers (hospitals and doctors) seeking to maximize profit (even if they are "not-for-profit") by manipulating the rules of the system. The fault is that we have Rube Goldberg-type com-plex constructs put in place to encourage behavior by providers, and providers are figuring out ways to work the system to their benefit. Gain to one part of the system (i.e., insurers) is a loss to another (i.e., providers), who then take actions that benefit them. The overall loser is the patient. Bavley quotes an email from a board member of a hospital system to the chief financial officer that said "Let's be realistic. Employing physicians is not achiev-ing better cost, it's achieving better profit." This isn't the view of some rogue hospital, but, as Batalden's law would predict, it is the very value that our system is designed to achieve, profit. Notice what is missing in the tension between the question of cutting costs and raking in profit: hiring doctors with the aim of improv-ing health care doesn't get a mention.

That is not what our national health policy should be about. We need to put everyone in a single-payer system, such as Medi-care, so some patients are not "more desirable" than others. We need a health system that pays for health care in a straightforward manner and has regulations that limit profit as the main motive for insurers, drug and device manufacturers, and providers. And we need to have Medicare, or whichever system we devise that would cover everyone, pay for the appropriate level of care for every patient. Then doctors and hospitals would have no incentive to focus on whether to label a person's hospitalization as "admission" or "observation", or an outpatient visit as "hospital based" or "office based" because there would be no difference in the reimbursement. It can be done. It is done in Canada. It is done in some fashion in every other developed country. If we decide that the health of our people is more important than the profit of the health care industry, we can do it also.

A conference I attended included a showing and discussion of the excellent film *Escape Fire*.[35] The film addresses many problems in our health care system, including dysfunctional delivery systems, an emphasis on high-tech "rescue" care rather than prevention, and profit-seeking by insurers, providers, and drug and device makers. There is also a segment that features Safeway's program for employee wellness. For some reason, the leaders of the ensuing discussion chose that as the basis for their first question to the audience: "Does your employer encourage wellness?"

After people made a number of comments, I observed that this was not the main point of the film, which mostly addressed the need for system change. A medical student present indicated that he agreed with most of what I said but that there should be some "individual accountability." I replied that individuals who took poor care of themselves faced the ultimate accountability— they got sick and died sooner. Of course, we should encourage our patients to eat right and exercise and not smoke and drive carefully, just as we should ourselves. However, trying to get each individual to always do the right thing is an inefficient and generally ineffective way to solve structural problems. Few of us never speed, but over the last 30 years there has been a tremendous decrease in traffic-related deaths. The reduction is mainly due to safer roads and more safely designed cars, and very little of it from people driving more carefully.

In the field of occupational health and safety, behavior change is considered a weak third option after architecture and engineering. If there is a big window next to the factory floor where it is sometimes slippery, that is an architectural flaw because people can accidentally smash the glass and fall out; it shouldn't be there. But, if there is one, you can put a heavy mesh screen over it so that if people do slip, they don't go through the window; this is engineering. Telling everyone to always be careful and not slip is good advice, but not a very effective solution. And yet this is essentially what doctors do with their patients with social problems all the time. While in no way do I wish to excuse physicians from making decisions that are based on criteria other than the best health interest of their patients, trying to get every doctor to always do the right thing is as unlikely to be successful as trying to get every person to never overeat, exercise daily, never speed or drink to excess, or ever do anything that is not in their best health interests. It would be good if people always did, just as it would be good if health care providers were never motivated by money. But it is not going to happen; we need systemic solutions.

Of course, an additional consideration in emphasizing individual behavior change is that we are wont to focus on it mostly with people whose "bad" behaviors are different from our own, and people who seem to be different from ourselves. *We* may overeat and need to go on a diet, but *they* are obese and at fault for it. *We* may drink sometimes, maybe too much, but *they* are alcoholics, or drug addicts. *We* could do a little more exercise, but *they* don't care at all for exercise and its health benefits. *We* sometimes indulge in a piece of cake or a donut or two, but *they* only eat crap.

We are sometimes in a hurry and not as careful as we should be, but *they* are maniacs on the road.

And, of course, this we/they comparison is exacerbated because *they* often look different from us, are of a different race or culture. And very often they are poorer than we are (especially when we are physicians), and confront, on a daily basis, a lot of challenges we don't. Do they live in a "food desert" where the nearest grocery is too far to walk and they haven't access to a car? Or it is unsafe to walk, for food or for exercise? Have they got a job or any chance of getting a job? Or are they "lucky" enough to have 3 jobs, and no time to "work out"? Judging others is a popular pastime, but it is often done without adequate understanding, and it is rarely useful. We can and should encourage healthful behaviors and try to identify obstacles and help people overcome them, but we must also focus on the systemic changes that make health possible in a more efficient and effective way than expecting everyone to change their behavior. The airlines have done it. The car industry (dragged kicking and screaming) has done it. Can the health care system do so as well? This is not certain; there are strong forces opposing a change to a single-payer, health-focused system. It will not be easy and success is not certain. We can take heart from struggles in the past against great odds, against slavery, and segregation, and women's suffrage, but none of these was a "sure-fire" bet. It will take people committed to justice, and committed to the idea that our U.S. health system needs to be re-designed to get the results that it should be able to get, to recognize that other countries have done it and we can too. And work very hard at it.

Two leading family medicine leaders have made pithy comments regarding our health system that might serve as appropriate codas to this chapter. Richard Wender, MD, echoes the sentiments of Greek physician Alex Benos when he says "Using health care as a driver of corporate economics as opposed to a public good is the fundamental cause of our medical inflation." Lee Green, MD, an American who is now a family medicine leader in Canada, adds:

> *Having practiced most of my career in the U.S., and now practicing in Canada, the contrast is quite evident. The U.S. health care system is not designed to get you the care you need, it is designed to get you the care that someone can make a profit giving you. If you're poor and uninsured, that's none - no matter how much you need it. If you're well-insured, it's a lot - including quite a bit you don't need, and even some that is harmful.[36]*

This is a great expression of Batalden's Law. It is no way to run a business, or a health care system. Our health is too important.

References

1   Green, L. Personal communication

2   As quoted in Bavley, A. Medicine goes corporate as more physicians join hospital payrolls. *K C Star*, December 28, 2013.

3   Benos, A. Personel communication.

4   Collins J. *How the Mighty Fall, And Why Some Companies Never Give In.* Collins Business Essentials, Harper Collins Books. 2009.

5   Schroeder, S., As quoted in Rosenthal, E. Health care's road to ruin, *New York Times.* December 21, 2013.

6   Kaplan, T. Bloomberg predicts fair deal if health insurer gets for-profit status, *New York Times,* Dec 23, 2011.

7   Rosenthal, E. The $2.7 trillion medical bill: colonoscopies explain why U.S. leads the world in health expenditures, *New York Times,* June 1, 2013.

8   Ibid #7.

9   Ibid #7.

10   A doctor's office that's all about you, *Consumer Reports,* July 2013.

11   Creswell, J, Meier, B. McGinty, JC. New Jersey hospital has highest billing rates in the nation. *New York Times,* May 16, 2013.

12   Rosenthal, E. After surgery, surprise $117,000 medical bill from doctor he didn't know. *New York Times* (complete ref)

13   Center for Medicare and Medicaid Services, Medicare provider charge data, http://www.cms.gov/Research-Statistics-Data-and-Systems/Statistics-Trends-and-Reports/Medicare-Provider-Charge-Data/index.html

14   Meier B, McGinty JC, Creswell J, Hospital billing varies wildly, government data shows, *New York Times,* May 8, 2013.

15   Chen C and Pearson S, Top medicare doctor paid $21 million in 2012, data show, *Bloomberg News,* April 9, 2014.

16   Gawande, A, The cost conundrum, *New Yorker,* June 1, 2009.

17   Brill, S, Bitter Pill: Why medical bills are killing us, *Time,* April 4, 2013.

18   Sibelius, K. As quoted by *Reuters Update.* U.S. Makes data available on wide-disparity in hospital charges. May 8, 2013.

19   Welch, HG, Diagnosis: insufficient outrage, *New York Times,* July 4, 2013.

20   Wise L, Medicare anti-fraud effort has Missouri roots, *Kansas City Star,* May 7, 2013.

21   Virchow, R, as quoted in Donohou, M, Schiff, GD. A call to service: Social justice is a public health issue. *Virtual Mentor* 16 (9): 699-707, September 2014.

22   Ibid # 2.

23   Ibid # 19.

24 Tilburt JC et al., Views of U.S. physicians about controlling health care costs, *JAMA* 310 (4): 380-389. 2013.

25 Emanuel EJ, Steinmetz A, Will physicians lead on controlling health care costs?, *JAMA* 310 (4): 374-5, July 24, 2013.

26 Ibid # 2.

27 Creswell J, Fink S, and Cohen S, Hospital charges surge for common ailments, data shows, by *New York Times,* June 2, 2014.

28 Editorial. The risks of hospital mergers, *New York Times*, July 6, 2014

29 Reuben DB, Cassel CK, Physician stewardship of health care in an era of finite resources, *JAMA* 306 (4): 430-1, July 27, 2011.

30 *Healthy People 2020.* http://www.healthypeople.gov/2020/default.aspx

31 Moriates C, Shah NT, Arora VM, First, do no (financial) harm, *JAMA.* 310 (6): 577-578, 2013.

32 Bettigole C, The thousand-dollar Pap smear, *N Engl J Med* 369(16): 1486-7, October 17, 2013.

33 Ibid # 32

34 Bavley, A, Facility fees' add billions to medical bills, *Kansas City Star,* December 30, 2013.

35 *Escape Fire: The fight to rescue American health care.* http://escapefiremovie.com/

36. Green, Lee. As cited by Wender, R, in a comment on a blog by Freeman, J, The high cost of US health care: it's not the colonoscopies, it's the profit.

Chapter 10

Designing a System to
Get the Results We Should Want

*Health and health care are not commodities that exist to
drive the economy. They are among the social goods that we
have an economy in order to be able to achieve.*[1]

—Alex Benos, M.D. Speaker at Physicians for a National
Health Program meeting, San Fransisco, 2012

*...the nation is fundamentally handicapped in its quest for
cheaper health care: All other developed countries rely on a
large degree of direct government intervention, negotiation
or rate-setting to achieve lower-priced medical treatment
for all citizens.*[2]

—Elisabeth Rosenthal, *New York Times*

The health care system in the U.S. is a train wreck. It is not
because of "flawed" design, but because of flawed goals. It is
well-designed (by definition) to get the results that it gets. These
come at a huge cost to us all, huge profits for some, and inferior
health outcomes for most Americans compared to other developed
countries. The system does not need tinkering or adjustments; it
does need a firm decision about what we want it to achieve, and a
redesign that will get us there.

Our system, in addition to costing so much and having relatively poor health outcomes, is inequitable and unjust. As I have discussed, it is focused on medical care rather than health, and preferentially on medical care for conditions that lend themselves to the most expensive, interventive treatments. It is not based on a firm foundation of primary care, as are most effective health systems. It is based on making profits, and many of the controversies and conflicts we read about are between providers and insurers over who is making the most. Finally, the most important determinants of health are outside of and come before interaction with the medical care, or even any aspect of the health care, system. They include the economic status of your family and of your family of origin. They include housing, food, education, warmth, discrimination, environmental pollution, and a host of other negative impacts that, in Dr. Camara Jones' analogy, put some people closer to the cliff face, more likely to fall off and then be at the mercy of whatever the medical care system does or does not provide.

However, even people who acknowledge that these disparities, inequalities and inequities exist, and that our health system is sorely deficient, do not always agree on what the most important problems actually are. Even when we eliminate overtly political posturing and consider only the honestly conceived beliefs of different players in the system, there is lack of consensus because there are many different perspectives from which to view the elephant of health care. In addition to these differences, there are differences in incentives, because what may be financially good for one part of the system is bad for others. Physicians and other individual providers, hospitals and health systems, politicians, policy makers and pundit—and of course patients—have different viewpoints. And, while there certainly is plenty of blame to go around and no shortage of people that any of us can point fingers at as the "real" problem, there is a solution: creating a system based on those that already exist in the world which lead to better health at lower cost.

There are many players in our health system, each seeing the others, rather than the system, as the problem. Physicians feel that they have an onerous regulatory burden and feel great pressure from their employers to see more patients rather that to provide high-quality care. The number of people who need care is increasing, in part from the one-time bolus of people getting health coverage under ACA, but more from a growing and aging population. There are exceptions to these generalizations: there are microsystems in the U.S. where care is capitated, where physicians and other providers (especially those in primary care) are organized into teams and paid on the basis of providing comprehensive care for individuals and populations, but these remain exceptions and are far from the norm in this country. From the perspective of most providers, efforts to increase access have increased their workload, decreased their job satisfaction, and, possibly most important, decreased their sense that they are providing quality health care to their patients.

Hospitals and health systems have built enormous physical plants and infrastructures based upon the "product lines" that are highly reimbursed (and, more important, have a high return on investment, or high reimbursement-to-cost-of-providing-the-service ratio), and they feel challenged by proposed changes in what is reimbursed. Like physicians, hospitals would like the public to think that they are in the business of delivering quality health care, but their emphasis, whether they are for-profit or non-profit, is often on the purely "business" part of their business. Policy makers, politicians, and pundits all have their own set of beliefs and interests which color their opinions.

Of course, there is the patient, who is ostensibly the focus of all the attention, for whom the entire health system is supposed to exist, but who is usually the least powerful player in the entire equation. Patients do not have the massive resources of hospitals and insurance companies. They do not have the medical knowledge of doctors. They are hopeful that their health will be the priority for those providing care, rather than some other set of interests, but cannot be certain of this. They may well not be able to pay for their care, or be bankrupted by trying. And, of course, there is not *a* patient, there are many individuals with different sets of needs and preferences.

In Chapter 5, I mention the article that Elisabeth Rosenthal wrote for the *New York Times* after a year of reporting on the crisis in health care, "Health Care's Road to Ruin."[3] That title pretty well describes where our current health system is headed. Ms. Rosenthal summarizes highlights from her investigations that looked at the extremely high cost of health care in the U.S. compared to other countries, the extreme variability in pricing depending upon where you are in the U.S., the opaque and incomprehensible methods of coming up with pricing, and the regulatory incentives that are continually gamed by providers. She then summarizes both the poor health outcomes at a population level in the U.S. compared to other countries, and the more personal, poignant and dispiriting stories of individuals who die, are bankrupted, or both by our health "system." The stories she tells, she notes, could be "Extreme anecdotes, perhaps. But the series has prompted more than 10,000 comments of outrage and frustration—from patients, doctors, politicians, even hospital and insurance executives."

This is very important, because it goes beyond the qualitative (there are many sad stories) to the quantitative—10,000 is a lot of people to write in and comment. First, it suggests that her anecdotes represent something widespread, not extreme. Second, it suggests that, whether the industry is ready for change or not, many people want something done and are frustrated enough to write about it. People are aware that the health system does not serve them or their interests. It begins to answer the question about whether Americans are ready for change: it suggests that the answer is "yes."

Rosenthal goes on to discuss the potential solutions that those commenters, and others, have suggested. These include: regulating prices, making medical schools cheaper or free, not paying fee-for- service that rewards volume rather than quality. But, she says,

> *...the nation is fundamentally handicapped in its quest for cheaper health care: All other developed countries rely on a large degree of direct government intervention, negotiation or rate-setting to achieve lower-priced medical treatment for all citizens. That is not politically acceptable here.*[4]

Well, it hasn't happened here, and it clearly has not been acceptable to our politicians, but her work and the response to it shows that it may well be acceptable to most Americans.

The Affordable Care Act

Before we move on to further discussion about such a truly new system, it is worth reviewing the Affordable Care Act (ACA), passed in 2010, the most extensive modification to health insurance in the U.S. since Medicare and Medicaid in 1965. Although far from the comprehensive redesign of the U.S. healthcare system that I think is necessary, the partial reforms contained in the ACA were loudly attacked by opponents of the program, and all of its early failings (such as its website) were widely publicized in the media. But, quietly, and with much less publicity, people signed up for ACA. In addition to the early benefits, such as allowing parents to keep their children on their insurance policy until the age of 26 and forbidding insurance companies to deny coverage to those with pre-existing conditions, ACA has dramatically expanded coverage, particularly in states that have opted for Medicaid expansion. Most of those now covered were either previously uninsured or pay much less than they had before. As noted earlier, people whose incomes are less than 133% of the poverty level were intended to be covered by Medicaid expansion; since the Supreme Court decision made participation in this program by states voluntary, we have seen far greater expansion in coverage in those states (just over half) that have opted to take part. As described by Paul Krugman in his piece "Obamacare fails to fail", July 14, 2014,

...people in the media—especially elite pundits—may be the last to hear the good news, simply because they're in a socioeconomic bracket in which people generally have good coverage....For the less fortunate, however, the Affordable Care Act has already made a big positive difference.[5]

People care about their health, and want to be able to access health care. The insurance exchanges set up by ACA, notwithstanding the attacks on them, are not government health insurance; they are government-supported private health insurance. The government is even prohibited from offering a "public option", but rather is depending upon insurance companies, motivated by their own profit opportunities, to provide coverage.

The political need is for the wealthy and powerful. This is why ACA ensured that insurance companies would get their cut. Elisabeth Rosenthal does not say this in so many words, but in her December 2013 article, with ACA partially implemented, she does say that:

> ...*after a year spent hearing from hundreds of patients...I know, too, that reforming the nation's $2.9 trillion health system is urgent, and will not be accomplished with delicate maneuvers at the margins. There are many further interventions that we know will help contain costs and rein in prices. And we'd better start making choices fast.* [6]

A universal health care program, "Medicare for all," in which everyone is automatically enrolled just as current Medicare recipients are now, would be a great first step.

In our current situation, there is already a shortage of physicians, mainly but not exclusively primary care physicians; the fact that under ACA, and in particular with Medicaid expansion (for those states actually expanding Medicaid) there will be more people with insurance and therefore more with access that will exacerbate this shortage. For example, a *New York Times'* lead article in November 2013 was "Medicaid growth could aggravate doctor shortage."[7] This implies that the doctor shortage is perceived to be worsened because there will be an increase in the number of people who have health insurance (from Medicaid expansion or insurance exchanges or any other reason). This is a callous misrepresentation. The shortage was already there because the people were already there, already needing to see doctors. They just didn't have the access. The reason that it was not perceived earlier was because people, not having health insurance, did not seek care. To the extent that they were not getting health care because they were uninsured was a scandal. If anything, the increase in coverage unmasks an unmet need.

The *Times* article focuses particularly on Medicaid because many doctors already will not see Medicaid patients since the payments are not high enough to cover their costs. Or, in many cases, it's because they can fill their schedules with people who have better-paying health insurance. This makes sense from a systemic perspective: when insurance pays some multiple of what the government pays, doctors are incentivized to shun Medicaid. It's built right into the system. Those physicians who do accept Medicaid often feel that they will not be able to take more Medicaid patients for the same reason, and it is unlikely that those who are already not accepting Medicaid will begin to do so. The problem is significant for primary care, even for institutions like Los Angeles' White Memorial Hospital that already care for large numbers of Medicaid patients. Hector Flores, Chair of the Family Medicine Department at White Memorial, notes in the same *New York Times* article that his group's practice already has 26,000 Medicaid patients and simply does not have capacity to absorb the potential 10,000 more that they anticipate will obtain coverage in their service area.

The problem in terms of gaining access to subspecialists may be even greater. There are already limited numbers of specialists caring for Medicaid patients in California and elsewhere, for the reasons described above: they have enough well-insured patients, and Medicaid (Medi-Cal in California) pays poorly. It is also possible that some subspecialists have less of a sense of social responsibility and feel no compunction to care even for a small number of patients who have Medicaid or are uninsured, and their expectations for income may be higher. The San Diego ENT physician featured at the start of the *Times* article, Ted Mazer, is one of the relatively small number of subspecialists who do take Medicaid, but indicates that he will not be able to take on more patients because of the low reimbursement.

Clearly, Dr. Mazer and Dr. Flores' group are not the problem, although it is likely that they will bear a great deal of the pressure under Medi-Cal expansion because their practices have already been accepting Medicaid; they are likely to be seen as the places to go when more people have Medicaid. The Beverly Hills subspecialists (such as those featured as the "Best Doctors" in any airline magazine—which in no way measures quality but simply means that they take care of the richest people) who have never seen Medicaid, uninsured, or poor people up until now, are unlikely to find them walking into their offices. And, if they call, they likely will not schedule them.

The real problem is that we have a health care system that is designed to make profit rather than improve health; this is the core issue that needs to be addressed in health system change, and must remain our focus. Many players within the system, however, do not take a holistic or comprehensive point of view, but see the world more narrowly based on their self-interest. From the point of view of doctors, or the health systems in which they work, the problem is inadequate reimbursement. A practice has to pay the physicians and the staff; if they work for salaries, the system they work for needs to make money to pay them. The *Times* article on Medicaid expansion notes that community clinics may be able to provide primary care, but does not note that many of them are Federally-Qualified Health Centers (FQHCs) which receive much higher reimbursement for Medicaid and Medicare patients than do other providers. The Affordable Care Act (ACA) will reimburse primary care providers an enhanced amount (10%) for Medicaid for two years, through 2014, but in many cases has yet to be put into place, and there is no assurance that this will continue. The specialists are not receiving this enhanced reimbursement, although—and because—many of them already receive significantly higher reimbursement for their work than primary care physicians.

If, however, we were to implement a single payer system, it would have an enormous impact on these reimbursement issues, in that it would free up a huge percentage of our GDP that could be used for raising payments if they are too low, and it would align doctors behind pushing the one payer to pay fairly. In such a situation, it would be easy for patients to organize in favor of getting their docs paid well—since a raise would not come out of their pockets and it is in their interest to have docs who are not under financial stress.

From a larger system point of view, Medicaid pays poorly because those opposed to Medicare and Medicaid have succeeded in restricting payments. (Although, as far as state expenditures are concerned, the federal government will pay 100% of the expansion for 4 years and 90% after that.) However, they do not want to be perceived as allowing lower quality of care for the patients covered by Medicaid, so they often add requirements for quality that increase costs to providers. This, in turn, increases the resistance of those already reluctant to accept it. Another very important factor is that Medicaid has historically not covered all poor people; rather it mainly covers young children and their mothers, a generally low-risk group. (It also covers nursing home expenses for poor people, which consume a much larger portion of its budget.) Expansion of Medicaid to everyone who makes 133% of the poverty level, as mandated by ACA (but not being implemented in nearly half our states) means that childless adults, including middle-aged people under 65 who have chronic diseases but have been uninsured, will now have coverage.

While the main impact of Medicaid expansion is in states like California that actually have expanded the program, even in states which have not, Medicaid enrollment has gone up because of all the publicity, which has led people who were already eligible but not enrolled to become aware of their eligibility (called, by experts, the "woodwork effect"). Because the structure of the ACA relies on the concurrent implementation of a number of different programs, Medicare reimbursements have been cut, as have "disproportionate share" (DSH) payments to hospitals providing a larger than average portion of unreimbursed care. This was supposed to have been made up for because formerly uninsured people would be covered by Medicaid (that is, hospitals would get something); however, with the requirement for that piece removed, thanks to the Supreme Court decision and the political beliefs of governors and state legislatures, the whole operation is unstable. Medicare and DSH payments will go down without compensatory increases in Medicaid, and hospitals are taking the financial hit.

At its core, the problem is not that the whole system is

flawed, but it is a complex monstrosity succeeding in what it was designed to do, make profits for some. While the ACA will help many more people, it is incomplete and is dependent on a lot of parts to work correctly and complementarily. As illustrated by the failure of many states to expand Medicaid, this does not always happen. A rational system would be one in which everyone was covered, and where reimbursements were at the same rates, so that lower reimbursement for some patients did not discourage providers from seeing them. These are not innovative ideas. These systems exist, in one form or another in every developed country: single payer in Canada, National Health Service in Britain, multi-payer private insurance with set costs and benefits provided by private non-profit insurance companies in Switzerland, and a variety of other arrangements in France, Germany, Taiwan, the Scandinavian countries, and others.

If payment to providers were the same for everyone that they care for, empowered people would ensure that it was adequate. Payment should be either averaged over the population or tied to the complexity of disease and treatment. We would have doctors putting most of their work into the people whose needs were greatest, rather than those whose ratio of reimbursement to difficulty of care ratio was highest. We need to move to a system that treats *people*, not "insurees", a system that is fair in its payment of doctors and other providers so that they can focus their efforts on treating people, not finding "insurees."

What Should Our Health System Be?

The data presented in Chapter 2 detailing the lower cost and better health outcomes in other OECD countries demonstrate that every other Western democracy has a better solution. And every one of them came through significant political struggle. They do it in different ways, probably reflecting the issues that existed for them when they had those political struggles, but the bottom line is that they cover everyone. Britain has a National Health Service, which contracts with physicians and owns hospitals, although they allow private insurance which a relatively small percent of the population has. Closest to us—in Canada—they have a single-payer system, essentially putting everyone into Medicare (Canada even calls its system Medicare). Other countries, such as France and Germany and Norway and Sweden and the Netherlands have different variations to choose among, should it turn out that we insist upon a more complex structure. Switzerland, for example, has multiple private insurance companies rather than a single payer, but they are highly regulated and non-profit; they are told by the government what they can charge and what they must cover. They compete for customers (patients) based on customer service. Key features of such a system are no private insurance and truly non-profit hospitals.

I would argue that the simplest and most efficient is a Canadian-style single payer system. This concept has been endorsed by a wide variety of experts, including those in business who pay for health insurance. This is the least complex and most cost effective way to do it. We would all be insured by the same system. We would all pay into that system while the government covers the bills. Providers could provide care to people based upon their disease, not their insurance status, and rates could be set at the level that we as a people are able to tolerate, or are willing to pay, for the health care we want and need. The clout of the empowered would bring along benefit for everyone. There would be no more incentive to favor patients based upon insurance status.

Unlike the British system, in Canada no private insurance is allowed for services that are provided by the provinces through Canadian Medicare. Since it is a province-by-province system, there is some variation in what those are. However, all 13 programs must provide the five key characteristics stipulated by the federal law that created it—they must be publicly administered, comprehensive, universal, portable (i.e., residents of one province must be covered in other provinces), and accessible. "Comprehensive" means that it covers all necessary inpatient and outpatient medical care, including mental health and dental care, so the uncovered areas that exist are generally in what we sometimes call "complementary and alternative" medicine (and most of these are covered as well), or in truly cosmetic procedures. Everyone in Canada is in. There are no people who are without health care coverage.

In the U.S., the huge number of insurers, both government (Medicare and Medicaid, as well as Tricare for military families and retirees) and private insurance companies, and the panoply of different "products" they offer, make billing and collecting a nightmare for providers. Someone has to figure out not only who the patient's insurer is, but which plan they have, what their co-pay is, whether they have met their deductible, and whether they have more than one and which is primary. Someone needs to appeal the decisions of the insurers to deny payment or pay incompletely. This has created an entire industry of healthcare billing and collecting, and professional billers. Huge U.S. teaching hospitals employ hundreds of people in the billing department, and every U.S. physician needs to employ a billing company, or if part of a large group, a cohort of billers, while comparable Canadian hospitals have a couple of people—mainly in case an insured American happens in, and doctors simply submit their bill to the single payer. The overhead cost in the U.S. system is enormous, and it is dramatically reduced in Canada.

What might be objections to the implementation of a Canadian-type single payer system? How about lost income and jobs?

The enormous cost of our U.S. health system, while not buying us better health, is buying something. The system that we have, after all, is perfectly designed to get the results that it gets. As discussed in the last chapter, many players—including insurance companies, providers, and drug and device manufacturers—are making big profits. They do not want to give this up. And, of course, there are the people employed by the industry in jobs that are not about actually providing health care, for example, all those billers and insurance salespeople. They would no longer be needed, and no one wants to lose a job. However, they are a weak reason to maintain our system. There are plenty of other jobs that need to be done, including those in providing health and social services that are currently underfunded; money saved on nonproductive healthcare administrative costs could begin to pay for some of these.

What about the fact that it is government healthcare, and the inefficiency that government has? Won't we have decreased efficiency, more faceless bureaucracy?

For starters, a single payer system is not government run health care, but government *paid* health care. In Canada, most doctors are in private practice or groups, and they are reimbursed by the single-payer on a fee for service basis, at rates negotiated annually between the medical societies and the provincial health ministries. This is not government-run health care, but government health insurance. It also means that Canada has some of the problems of fee-for-service that I will discuss. Some hospitals are government owned, as in the U.S., but most are private nonprofits, as they are here. The difference is that they operate on a global budget negotiated with the health ministry. Importantly, capital costs (new buildings, buying major new equipment such as MRI scanners) are budgeted separately, so that the hospitals are not motivated to skimp on care in order to save money for capital expenses.

The U.S. government actually does a pretty good job of paying for things; people get their Social Security checks, and Medicare pays their bills. Indeed, during the debate on the Affordable Care Act, we often heard people say "keep the government's hands off my Medicare!" Humorously ironic, perhaps, but it is also an indication of how much people actually value the government programs that provide benefit to them. And faceless bureaucracy? Anyone who has tried to complain to their health insurance company about a bill knows how difficult it is to even get in touch with them, not to mention receive satisfaction. Nearly half of all health care expenses are already paid by governments (Medicare, Medicaid, Tricare, military, veterans, employees and retirees from federal, state and local governments), and if the tax breaks that employers (but not employees) get for their contributions to their employees' health insurance is counted, it is more than half.

But Medicare doesn't pay that well, and Medicaid pays even worse. Won't this make our health care worse? What about waits for procedures in other countries such as Canada and Britain?

It is true that reimbursement to providers from publicly funded programs is less than it costs in some cases to provide the care, particularly from Medicaid. Some of this would be addressed by a single payer simply because the overhead costs would go down, so the cost of care would be less; "health care costs" would mainly be for actually providing care. The more important issue is separating how much money is spent on health care and how that money is distributed. In most countries, everyone is covered, but sometimes the total amount budgeted is too little, and needs to be increased. In Britain, for example, wait times were getting so long that there was dissatisfaction among people, and enough complaints (and elections) occurred that funding for the NHS was increased. Now, on average, people wait less than in the past for most necessary procedures, and the cost per capita, while higher, is still far less than in the U.S. The main important point, as I will continue to reiterate, is that everyone is in the same system. Unlike in the U.S., where some people are on Medicaid or Medicare, and others have a variety of high to low quality private insurance, and yet others are uninsured, everyone has the same coverage. Thus, everyone has an incentive to make sure that the system is adequately funded to meet their health needs; the voices of the more influential mean that the care given to the powerless is still improved.

But is this American? What about competition?

Can competition drive down prices in health care? This is certainly one argument that has been put forward for competition in health care—that it prevents artificially inflated charges and cost, just as it sometimes does in other parts of the marketplace. The answer is most obviously positive in price-sensitive elective care. In a widely-seen interview with John Oliver on "The Daily Show", Senator Rand Paul of Kentucky, an ophthalmologist, tried to demonstrate the benefit of competition and how the "market" controls costs by referring to how it led to big price drops for two major procedures in his specialty, Lasik® surgery and contact lenses.[8] With regard to the former, he notes that competition among ophthalmologists has led to dramatic decreases in charges from over $2,000 an eye to less than $500. The competition for contact lenses was with large retailers like Wal-Mart, which forced him to drop his charges in order to compete. Neither was covered by insurance, but he uses them as examples of how this could work for other things that *are* covered by insurance and to which people are price-insensitive.

Could Senator Paul be correct, then, that competition is the way to go? The cost of both Lasik® and contact lenses have indeed dropped, but the reason is that these are both elective procedures that generally are not covered by insurance, and thus (like cosmetic surgery and many consumer items) can be reasonably subject to market forces. There is a cheaper and effective option that works for the medical problem: glasses. If you are considering Lasik® or contact lenses, you can choose to not buy them now and wait until prices come down. However, most of healthcare is not elective, but is more like food and housing. Emergencies are emergencies and need to be addressed fast, by the most available provider.

Family physician and evidence-based medicine expert Mark Ebell notes a more apt comparison: "If you have a stick in your eye, I doubt that you are price shopping or waiting for ads on the radio to advertise a special for removal of sticks in the eye."[9] You bet! And while not all necessary healthcare is about such emergencies, most of it is not about elective procedures either. Chronic diseases like hypertension and diabetes need to be treated in order to prevent their progression to serious outcomes. Preventive care like screening for cancer and immunizations are only of value if they happen before the onset of disease. Neither Lasik® nor contact lenses prevent disease or its progression, and as such are good examples of elective, price-sensitive health care for which the market works, but they are not the typical reasons people seek medical care. Indeed, the importance of competition is most obvious when it is absent and prices rise for needed and even emergent services, as demonstrated in the case of hospitals that have a lock on their market.

While business leaders often extol the benefits of competition, in fact most would prefer to have such a "lock," a monopoly on the market (or at least be part of an oligopoly, where only a few players exist in a market and often collude on pricing) as it maximizes their profit. Airfares are a good example; I live in Kansas City, and if I fly to NYC, the round-trip fare for a non-stop is more than twice what it is to fly to Washington, D.C. This was not always true; there used to be several airlines flying non-stop from

KC to NY, but now there is one, while there are at least 2 flying to DC. So, NYC costs more because there's no competition.

Many of our core services are delivered non-competitively by government: police and fire are two of the many that come to mind. We do this because we believe that they are social goods which everyone should share in, and should be paid for collectively, by tax money. When your house is on fire, and the fire department comes, it takes care of it as best it can; it dosen't look to see what type of insurance you have. Most other countries have decided that healthcare is a similar social good, and pay for it publicly. We should as well.

Health Information Technology: a Helpful Tool Or a Real Solution?

Health information technology is a prime example of the tension between coordination and competition. Heavily encouraged and subsidized by the federal government as a way to improve coordination of care, technology such as electronic health records (EHRs) can in theory promote both competition and coordination, but only if they are implemented well. An interoperable health information technology (IT) environment, for example, should promote both, but health IT without interoperability may simply lock patients in to their current providers or provider networks by making it difficult or costly to move their records, reducing competition. The opportunities for a win–win are limited.

Most providers who use EHRs will acknowledge their advantages ("I know what is happening elsewhere–at least within the system") but complain about the amount of time it takes to enter data. They also note that many large systems they work for have bought the components of systems that facilitate billing, but less often those that offer benefits for patient care, such as "registries" (lists of the patients with similar conditions, such as diabetes, who may need similar regular interventions). Interoperability does not exist. Provider lock–getting a healthcare system to spend so much money on your EHR product that they can't change–has become the *de facto* strategy for most health IT companies. "The worst nightmare of most health IT companies," says a friend who is an expert in the field, "is that Apple will get involved and create a product that works better and is easy to use. And will probably be cheaper. So they want to lock you in." Health information technology (HIT) has two different objectives: make records accessible to providers and streamline billing. The first is admirable, and is something both providers and patients want. But the second is a need largely because our private for-profit system is so complex. With hundreds of private insurers it is almost impossible to follow all the billing rules of each one. Single payer would remove that complexity—one payer, one set of rules—and makes this aspect of HIT archaic and unnecessary.

Much of the discussion of health IT, as often is the case in rarefied discussions of health policy, does not address the most important point: What is best for the health and health care of people, or patients? Not "consumers", those largely-hypothetical well-informed people whose problems are so non-urgent and budgets so large that they can shop for health care as they might for shoes, but the rest of us; people who are sick, who are stuck in their health plans (whether government like Medicare and Medicaid or because their employer only offers one) or are uninsured. To the extent that HIT improves quality of care by facilitating communication between providers, it is good for people. To the extent that it simply facilitates the tug of war between providers and insurers, it is simply a tool for working within an unjust system.

This is where doctors are often right when they talk about meddling by bureaucrats. Policies adopted by Medicare and private insurers to attempt to influence both quality and cost are often quite different from each other, but more to the point are indirect. They attempt to influence both the quality and cost of care by financial incentives or disincentives, and this permits—indeed encourages—gaming of the system, trying to maximize income while minimizing cost and risk. This is often detrimental to patients. The solution may well be more explicit regulation to directly address what needs to happen. Not micromanagement ("use this drug"), although following evidence-based treatment approaches should be among them, but policies that explicitly encourage high-quality, cost-effective care. Coordinate care, but block monopolies; encourage consolidation between organizations providing complementary rather than the same services; do not pay higher amounts because a system has a monopoly; legislate that health IT systems be interoperable; measure quality outcomes that control for severity of illness and the socioeconomic risk factors of patients.

A single-payer health system, Medicare-for-all, could have the clout to make this happen.

How about quality? And efficiency?

In previous chapters, I have addressed the distressing-but-true fact that there is frequently much lower quality in American health care than we would like to think. This is most apparent when looked at from a population perspective. But even from an individual point of view there are an unconscionably high rate of errors and avoidable complications, as well as problems that come from people delaying care due to cost and from the use of treatments that make someone money, but may not be effective. I have addressed the need for a healthcare system to have an adequate base of primary care, so that people can access the appropriate health care providers who can manage most of their conditions and act as their advocate.

Single payer is only a payment system; it is not a total re-design of our health care system to be focused on health rather than profit. But it provides the basis for taking the other actions needed to control costs, enhance quality, and provide more equitable access. In such a system, where activities are financed by a central payer, insurance company profit is no longer part of the system. This means that prices for treatments can be standardized, and costs can be transparent. It means a single entity that can set standards for care and quality across the board. It means that prices of drugs can be negotiated with manufacturers. Single payer does not require, for example, that payment for care be capitated rather than fee-for-service (indeed, in Canada most ambulatory care is paid on a fee-for-service basis) but it provides a strong foundation for an effective prospective payment system.

Even if we do stay with an FFS system, the single payer will have sufficient clout to regulate excessive or unnecessary care, and a wide enough constituency (all of us) to ensure that our resources are used for all of us, rather than too much care for some and too little for others. If, as could be anticipated, the cost of delivering quality care goes down through administrative cost savings and the elimination of large amounts of profit being taken out of the system, this money is now available to the government to spend on addressing the social determinants of health. When everyone is part of the same system, rather than just some of us in the Medicare single-payer system that exists for the aged, blind, and disabled, providers will be motivated to ensure that it pays sufficiently, rather than motivated to avoid the people it covers.

I have noted that for certain elective, non-critical medical interventions (such as the Lasik® and contact lenses mentioned by Senator Paul) the competitive market could drive down cost. A single-payer system would theoretically lose this advantage, since all services would be paid for by the same payer at the same rate. A single payer, however, does not mean a single provider of care. It is still possible to have differences of quality or other character-istics that might distinguish one vendor, differences that matter to people. Providers of services might compete, if they wished, on the basis of quality outcomes or personal style. But providers will not be able to charge more for these characteristics. People do not care about being able to choose their health insurance company, although they do want to have as comprehensive coverage as they can afford; under a single payer system, all of us would have the same comprehensive coverage, and all of us would be able to af-ford it. Once a single payer is paying all the bills in this way, there is no reason for a person to care about their insurer, to ago-nize over incomprehensible policies, to attempt to balance risk of one problem or another, to worry about lower monthly premiums for a high-deductible plan versus the potential for enormous cost if they fall ill. A major and unnecessary burden would be taken from people's lives; like the protagonists in Kaurismäki's film *Le Havre*, discussed in Chapter 3, they can worry about their health without worrying about the bills.

By far the most important point, however, is that if we are all in, if even the most privileged have the same coverage as everyone else, it will protect the interests of the most vulnerable better than any form of competition in the marketplace. The competition that exists now allows private companies to opt out of covering them, allows them to compete for only the best paying, lowest cost people and puts the poor and sick and old in a separate system in which others do not have a stake. When everyone uses the same system, there is a powerful voice for a well-funded system, because everyone depends on it to function well. Plus, everyone pays taxes to finance the system, so they are invested in its efficiency. Having such a system would certainly be evidence of a core commitment to social justice.

The cost of health care and how to decrease it are a recurring theme in the political arena, but our concern has to go beyond cost to using the money that is spent wisely and to greatest effect. We must emphasize the need to increase access to necessary health and medical care to all people who need it, and, even more, to create social conditions that decrease the burden of ill health. The ACA was in part designed to do both, but much of its focus has been on cutting costs.

In Chapter 4, I cited the work of Kangovi and colleagues who examined the reasons that poor people use hospital emergency rooms "inappropriately" for care, to the frustration of the ERs, primary care doctors, payers, and health policy experts.[10] The 3 major groups of reasons were quality (or, more accurately, perceived quality), cost (a matter not of overall cost but of out-of-pocket cost to the user at the time of service), and convenience (which I argue is a misleading word for describing a place that is actually open and will see you when you can get there).

It would be a serious mistake, however, to presume that it

is just the inappropriate use of health services by poor people that drives up the cost of care. Indeed, this is only a small part of the excess cost of health care in the U.S. I define "excess cost" as cost in excess of what would be needed to be provide quality care to everyone. Another way to define this excess cost is as the additional cost per capita spent in this country compared to many other developed countries whose health outcomes are much better than ours while costing less. Major reasons for our high administrative costs result from the war between providers and insurers about what will be paid for and how much. This requires enormous numbers of people on both sides. Profits are pulled from our system by investors as resources are directed, even by non-profits, to high-margin activities. All this would all be effectively eliminated in a single payer system. Yes, other drivers of excess cost, such as procedures that didn't need to be done, over-utilization of high-cost technology, under-utilization of primary care, and poor geographic distribution of medical care would not be automatically eliminated by single payer, but the infrastructure for addressing them would be in place; that is, a single payer system becomes a necessary, if not sufficient, mechanism for control of these costs.

If we are to design a new system that will get the results that we want to get, it will also be critical to address the fact that the U.S. does not provide anywhere near the overall social service safety net that other developed countries do. In those other countries there is much more spent to ensure that people have adequate food, housing, education, and a living wage, which are all drivers of health status. While these issues, addressed in Chapter 2, are outside the formal health system and so are not intrinsic to a single-payer system, they do share with such a system the fact that they are motivated by, and are indicators of a society committed to, justice and equity, a society that cares for its citizens. Both single-payer and addressing the social determinants of health would indicate a society that could meet the test of FDR for progress: "...not whether we add more to the abundance of those who have much. It is whether we provide enough for those who have little."

Whatever payment system exists, there will always be times when people are confronted with difficult decisions about what to do for themselves or their loved ones when they are sick or close to death. Do more? Will it help? How likely is it to help? What does "help" mean? Is cure possible? Is a meaningful life possible? If it does help, for how long is it likely to? Will the decision have to be made again next week, next month, next year? These are incredibly hard choices, but they do not have to be further complicated by cost. A single-payer in a rational system can remove this dimension from these decisions.

In Chapter 8, I wrote about former President George W. Bush receiving a cardiac stress test as part of his annual physical. This led to a CT angiogram and finally the placement of a stent in one of his coronary arteries. Rather than demonstrating what fine care the privileged get, it was an example of how getting too much care can be inappropriate or harmful even for the most privileged. The narrowed coronary artery was found because of a cascade of tests that are not recommended for an *asymptomatic* 67-year old man. The stent that was placed in a narrowed area of his coronary artery will not prevent further progression of any coronary artery disease. Such stents are of value if they relieve pain, but the President did not have pain; he was able to do extremely high levels of exercise for his age pain free. And while he apparently did not have any of the uncommon but real potential complications of stent placement, he will now have to be on two anti-platelet drugs.

Yet many doctors and hospitals will tell you that they have often recommended against interventions because they have little or no likelihood of meaningful benefit, and often a significant risk of harm, only to be told by the patient and/or family that they want to "do everything." Often these people suspect that if they had more money, or if they were a different color, or if they were in a "better" hospital, the providers wouldn't be suggesting that they forego further intervention. I don't doubt that this is sometimes justified, and I'm sure that if a patient has enough money to spend there will be someone, somewhere, whether "quack" or a "legitimate" medical center, who will take it to "do something." But this doesn't make it right or good. I have not seen formal studies but a number of anecdotes would suggest that many of those with the most resources are among those with the most unpleasant deaths. Our culture values intervention, and they have the money to find some who is willing to make a profit intervening.

In a moving and important essay, Ken Murray, himself a physician, describes "How doctors die."[11] It rings true with almost every doctor I know. What they want for themselves is to die in peace, without useless interventions. If only those we physicians care for, who might feel that they are being denied something, could know that is what we choose for ourselves. Americans will, sadly, be just as desperate to try one more thing under single payer as they are under the current one. So that aspect of unnecessary cost (and pain) won't diminish under single payer. But what will be absent is the additional concern that "if I had more money or better insurance they would be doing this for me, or my loved one", and that makes it much easier to believe that what is being recommended is in fact the best medical advice.

Everyone dies. We would all like, and like for our loved ones, to live as long as possible if our lives have meaning—some physical and/or intellectual function, some ability to contribute to or benefit from others. We would like, and like for our loved ones, to be comfortable and pain-free as we approach death. We don't want to think that money which could help us or our loved ones is being "saved" just so it can be used to provide services to others who are richer or louder, and certainly not so that insurance companies can make more profit. But when something will not "help" in any meaningful way, and may hurt, our providers should recommend that it not be done, and we should be able to trust that they are making these recommendations because they are truly in our best interests, not because someone will make more, or lose less money. Not doing is often more appropriate and more power-ful than doing. We must focus on doing the right thing, the best thing for patients, whether that is another procedure or support and pain relief. We cannot and should not have to put up with health care providers who advertise and promulgate interventions that are unproven, or will not help, or will harm, because they can make a profit doing it.

If we are to get to this place as a society, where the U.S. health care system is one designed to get you the care you need rather than to get you the care that someone can make a profit pro-viding to you, we are going to have, as a society, to indicate that this is a value we share. And that change of attitudes and behavior needs to start at the top of the social and economic scale, not at the bottom. No unnecessary stents for President Bush, no "execu-tive physicals", no inappropriate end of life interventions for the wealthy. A system in which the "best" in healthcare is not defined as the "most", but the most effective and most appropriate for the person at the time.

One recurrent theme of this book has been the importance of everyone having access to necessary medical care, and how the U.S. compares poorly to other developed countries in that it does not cover everyone. Another has been that many medical procedures are unnecessary, sometimes even harmful, but are nonetheless provided to people who have the money or insurance to pay for them. This is not to say that greed is always the motivator; there is a powerful, if often incorrect, belief that to do something is better than to do nothing. We have too many people with real needs not getting appropriate care to be spending money on inappropriate and potentially dangerous care for others.

The most ubiquitous argument for not expanding, or even cutting, social services, including health care for the most needy, is that we "cannot afford it." (There are other arguments, primarily ideological and often self-serving for the privileged, but these reasons will only convince those ideologues.) However, not having enough money, not being able to afford things, is something that the great majority of people can relate to because they know what it is to not have enough money, to not be able to afford things that they would like, and often things that they need. So the argument, though false, resonates with people. This, therefore, is the argument put forward by the governors and legislatures in states that have refused to expand Medicaid as part of the ACA. The clear and convincing evidence to the contrary that it will cost states much *more* not to expand it doesn't shake their faith.

The real reasons for opposing expansion are more likely ideological than a true worry about cost, and the desire of the incredibly rich and powerful to further expand their wealth and power, and the desire of elected officials to get money from the rich and powerful for their election campaigns. Nonetheless, the reason given to the public is that there is a lack of money. That the lack of money in the public sector is largely a result of ideologically-driven tax cuts that overwhelmingly benefit the rich and powerful is ironic. It is not lost on people; the "occupy" movement and the identification of the 1% as the "they" compared to the rest of us (although it is probably the 0.1% or an even smaller group with most of the money and power). Nonetheless, the idea that there is not enough money for "helping people" has gained great traction, especially with those who see themselves as middle-class and be-leaguered.

The key issue here is the degree to which such expenditures are seen as helping others rather than helping society, or even helping "ourselves." The expansion of coverage through insurance exchanges established by the ACA, though deeply flawed, helped lots of people who did not see themselves as the typical beneficiaries of government programs; indeed, many of the lowest income people are unable to get coverage because they are unlucky enough to live in states that have not expanded Medicaid. People do understand social programs that benefit them; they understand and support Social Security and Medicare, the most popular programs ever instituted by the American government,[12] because they are recipients themselves, or have family members that are, or they are likely to be recipients in the future. Those who see themselves as more "conservative" justify what they might otherwise characterize as "handouts" if paid to someone else by characterizing it as something that they have earned through their work.

In fact, the benefits from Social Security and Medicare Part A are primarily funded by current workers payments, and exceed what was paid in by recipients; all of outpatient Medicare (Part B) is paid from general tax revenues. There is nothing wrong with this, but the fact of it is often obscured by those who would have you believe that these are different from other government programs because you already paid for it, unlike other programs that will help "them." And, of course, many people are willing to accept largess for themselves even when it contradicts both the beliefs that they have and how they vote; this can be true of agricultural subsidies as well as subsidies for corporations and tax codes that tax the income of financiers as if it were capital gains (not to mention the taxing of capital gains at a lower level than income in the first place).

But expansion of health care to everyone, and more generally expansion of social services to improve the health status of everyone, is beneficial to the society. It creates a healthy workforce, it means people have the ability to contribute by their labor and spirit and taxes, to raise their children, to be vital and productive members of society. It is certainly not charity, especially when it is received by everyone. I think many people agree with this, and most polls show that the large majority of people support a universal health care system (although they may be suspicious of any particular one, including the ACA).[13] Moreover, most people, even those that do not agree in those polls, even those who live in "red" states, even those who see themselves as conservatives, are good and caring people who would and do help individuals, those they know and those they don't. When "Baby Jessica" fell down a well in Texas in 1987, regular people who didn't know her or her family, people from all over the country, sent tens of millions of dollars. People are caring.

But How Can We Afford It?

As I thought about this issue of cost, I happened to watch the first episode of the British television series "Call the Midwife." This story takes place in a different time, a different place, a different culture. Is there anything we can learn, I wondered, that could apply to us? Set in a poverty-stricken area of East London in 1957, midwives pedal their bicycles around the crowds of people and rubble that still covers the streets more than a decade after the end of World War II to attend to pregnant women in their homes, delivering prenatal care and babies and even caring for the babies afterward. It is a not a beautiful scenario; the young midwife, Jenny Lee (based on the real life midwife Jennifer Worth, whose memoirs form the basis for the series and who died in 2011) has never seen such poverty, such crowding, such filth, so many children. It is the height of the "baby boom", attributed initially to returning soldiers who had to wait to start their families, but continuing with no end in sight; the women portrayed are having their fourth or fifth baby in their early 20s and many having far more. In fact, of course, the end of this "boom" was not the aging out of the reproductive population but the introduction of effective and widely available contraception (especially birth control pills) in the 1960s.

The midwives, all nurses and many of them nuns, set up clinics in a gym in the interval between the pensioners' breakfast and the evening dance classes, as well as attending women at home. The obstetrics that they practiced is quaintly anachronistic today, but they provided much safer pregnancies and deliveries than had ever been available to this poor population in the past. A woman in dire straits after her delivery is cared for at home while they await the arrival of the "obstetrics flying squad" with its ambulance, obstetrician, and pediatrician to continue the care. When the mother refuses to send her premature baby to the hospital, the senior midwife tells Jenny that they will visit three times a day until the baby is stable, and then at least once a day thereafter. In the home.

It is a dramatic and engaging story, but what fascinates me is that while *Call the Midwife* may be fictionalized, these services were actually available to these poor women. Home visits for prenatal care and delivery. Visits from nurses three times a day. An obstetrics "flying squad" to come to the homes of women who would otherwise die in childbirth. Where did the money for these services come from? Who paid them? Surely, some credit can go to the order of nuns who were the original midwives for decades, but this is far from all of it. The young midwives who are not nuns are paid. And these flying squad doctors? Well, they were paid, and the services were (and are) provided by the National Health Service (NHS).

This somewhat alien (remote in time, but not in the existence of poverty) setting contains a powerful insight for those wondering if we can afford a single payer system in the U.S. The NHS was established after the World War II, in 1948, to provide health care to all people in the UK. It was not established at a time of prosperity, when they could "afford" it, but at a time when both the nation's economy and its infrastructure were literally in shambles. The piles of rubble were still on the streets of London in 1957, 15 years after the Blitz. The National Health Service was not founded at a time of plenty, or as a gesture of magnanimity from the wealthy, but as an explicit and well-thought out policy to provide one of the most basic of needs, health care, to all of the British people. Even though there was not much money; it was seen as a priority. In a later episode of *Call the Midwife*, a woman who has lost four babies because of a pelvis contracted from rickets (vitamin D deficiency in childhood) is delivered a healthy baby by Caesarean section. Rickets itself, the senior midwife says, is a disease of poverty and malnutrition that has been eliminated by the NHS.

Will we create a single payer system in the U.S.? We can't predict the answer. But at least we know it's not a matter of money. It's a matter of building the political will. And, in doing that, we all have a role.

References

1   Benos, A. Personal communication.

2   Rosenthal E., Health care's road to ruin, *New York Times*, December 21, 2013.

3   Ibid #2

4   Ibid #2

5   Krugman P, Obamacare fails to fail, *New York Times*, July 14, 2014.

6   Ibid #2

7   Goodnough A, Medicaid growth could aggravate doctor shortage, *New York Times*, November 28, 2013.

8   "The Daily Show", August 12, 2013. http://thedailyshow.cc.com/videos/bn48rb/rand-paul

9   Ebell, M. Personal communication.

10 Kangovi S, et al., Understanding why patients of low socioeconomic status prefer hospitals over ambulatory care , *Health Aff* vol. 32 no. 7 1196-1203, July, 2013.

11 Murray K, How doctors die, *J Miss State Med Assoc.* 54 (3): 67-9. March, 2013.

12   Taylor P, *The Next Generation: Boomers, Millennials, and the Looming Generational Showdown,* p. 15. Public Affairs, NY.

13   Sullivan K, Informative polls show two-thirds support for single-payer, posted on PNHP website, http://pnhp.org/blog/2009/12/09/two-thirds-support-3/ December 9, 2009

About the Author

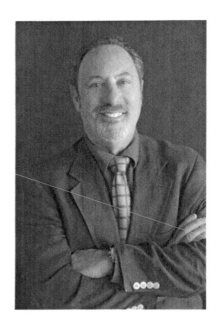

Joshua Freeman, M.D., is a physician educator and health and social justice activist. He serves as Alice M. Patterson, MD and Harold L. Patterson, MD Professor and Chair of the Department of Family Medicine at the University of Kansas Medical Center in Kansas City, where he is also Professor of Preventive Medicine and Public Health and of Health Policy and Management. He writes the widely-read blog *"Medicine and Social Justice"*. Dr. Freeman has recently served as a national officer of both the Society of Teachers of Family Medicine and the Association of Departments of Family Medicine, and is a Trustee of Roosevelt University in Chicago. He is the father of grown children, and lives in Kansas City, KS with his life partner, Patricia Kelly, and their dogs.

CPSIA information can be obtained at www.ICGtesting.com
Printed in the USA
BVOW03s2340210615

405041BV00003B/203/P

9 780988 799684